Sickle cell

A SCOPE® PUBLICATION

Marion I. Barnhart, Ph. D.
Professor of Physiology
Wayne State University School of Medicine
and
Director of Bargman Foundation Laboratory
for Cell and Molecular Research

Raymond L. Henry, Ph. D.
Professor of Physiology
and
Director of Graduate Program in Physiology
Wayne State University School of Medicine

Jeanne M. Lusher, M.D.
Professor of Pediatrics and
Director, Division Hematology and Oncology,
Children's Hospital of Michigan.

Upjohn

Herbert L. Gross
Editor

Larry L. Fites
Senior Art Director

Library of Congress Card Number 73-92193

S-3622-R1

CONTENTS

PREFACE

Sickle cell disease is the most common hereditary hematologic disorder known in man. Worldwide in distribution, it affects primarily Black Africans and Americans, as well as some Latins. It is estimated that in the United States alone some fifty thousand blacks have the severe form, sickle cell anemia.

Observations of sickle cell disease date back many years. As early as 1910 Herrick noted peculiarly shaped sickle cells in the peripheral blood of a Black West Indian student. However, the molecular era for the study of sickle cell disease did not begin until the identification of hemoglobin S as a molecular abnormality by Linus Pauling in 1949. Over the next two decades Max Perutz as well as other brilliant investigators made valuable contributions which ultimately led to the development of a molecular hypothesis for sickling of hemoglobin S erythrocytes by Makio Murayama in 1964. Based on Murayama's hypothesis, Robert Nalbandian and associates devised specific tests for the presence of hemoglobin S, as well as new treatment regimens. These, as well as additional regimens developed by others, are still in the investigational phase.

We are now in the midst of an exciting era of molecular research in sickle cell disease. While there have been many significant advances in our understanding of this condition within the past few years, many challenges must still be met.

This monograph is designed to give the medical student, house officer, and practitioner up-to-date information regarding various aspects of sickle cell disease. Included are descriptions of the abnormal molecule, of molecular mechanisms involved in sickling, of structural physiology of Hb SS erythrocytes and the microcirculation, of methods of testing and screening, and of clinical manifestations and treatment. It is hoped that you, the reader, will become sufficiently interested to meet the challenges that remain!

Figure 1. This model represents one molecule of hemoglobin S magnified 127 million times (scaled to ½ inch per angstrom). There are 10 thousand atoms in the molecule. Hb S is composed of 4 polypeptide chains; the upper half represents 2 α chains, each containing 141 amino acid residues. The lower half of model depicts 2 β chains, each with 146 amino acid residues. The only difference between Hb S and Hb A (normal) is that valine is substitued for glutamic acid in each β chain.

For identification of atoms the color code follows: red=oxygen, white=hydrogen, blue=nitrogen, yellow=sulfur, silver=carbon.

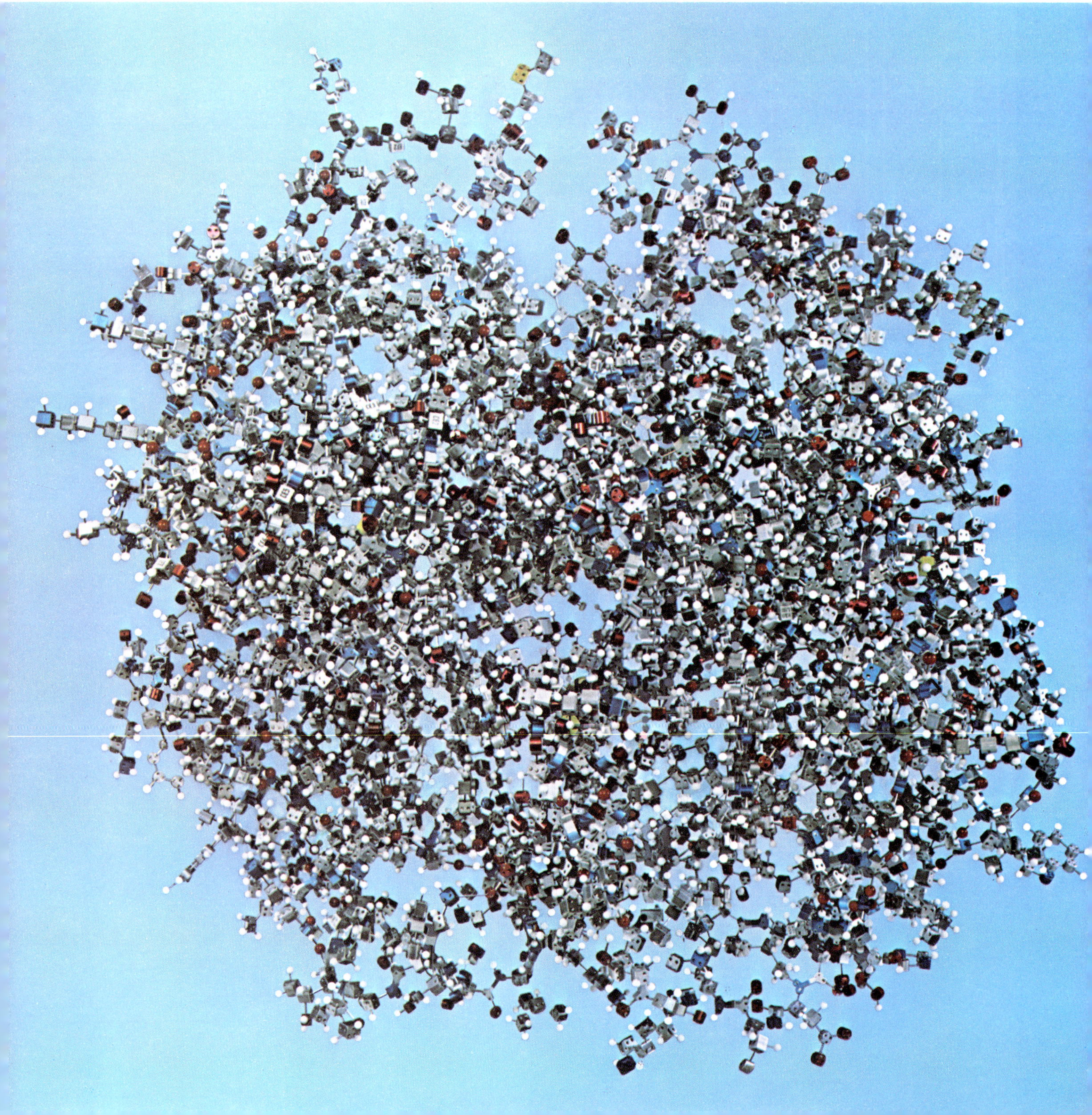

The Disease

Sickle cell disease is a genetic disorder characterized by an abnormal hemoglobin molecule, designated hemoglobin S (Fig. 1) which can distort erythrocytes (RBC) into sickle cells (Fig. 2). While some reserve the term "sickle cell disease" for the homozygous state (SS) only, others use it in a broader or generic sense to include *all* conditions in which hemoglobin S is present. By the latter definition the sickle cell disease states would include not only sickle cell anemia (SS), but also the usually benign "carrier" state (AS), doubly heterozygous hemoglobinopathies (as SC, SD) and S-thalassemia.

Sickle cell disease is a world-health problem predominantly affecting Negroes in the United States and Africa and to a lesser extent Latins, and selected populations generally adjacent to the Mediterranean Sea and Indian Ocean. The sickle cell gene, an autosomal recessive, is passed on to both male and female children. It is essential to recognize that gene expression and the course of the disease are variable, governed by the exact inheritance and interaction with environmental factors.

Sickle cell anemia is a disease of serious proportions. It is characterized by a chronic hemolytic anemia, recurrent attacks of pain, frequent bacterial infections, gradual deterioration of tissue and organ function and a shortened life expectancy. While no accurate statistics are available at present, reasonable estimates are that the homozygous state afflicts one in 500 Black children within the United States, or 50,000 of the nation's 22 million Blacks.

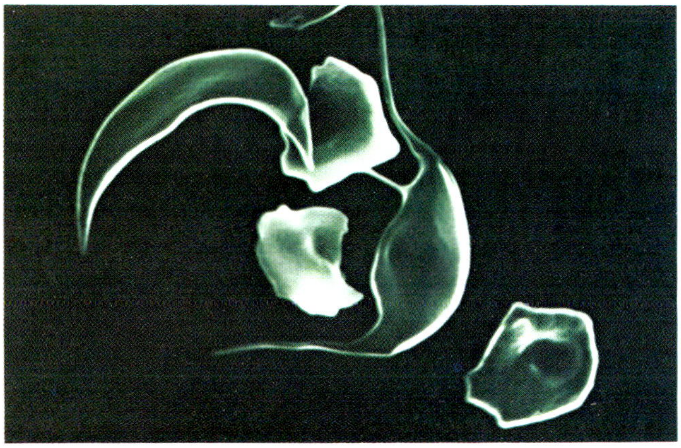

Figure 2. Scanning electron micrograph (SEM) of sickled RBC, deoxygenation induced with sodium metabisulfite, from a Hb SS individual (X 6600).

The heterozygous state, sickle cell trait, is benign under ordinary physiologic conditions but is important primarily from a genetic standpoint. Some two million American Blacks (8-10%) have sickle trait. If two such "carriers" mate, their offspring will have a one-in-four chance of having the severe form of the disease, sickle cell anemia.

Although recognized since 1910, sickle cell disease has risen from relative obscurity to national prominence within the past six years. Within this period, federal funding for research, detection, genetic counselling, education, and clinical trials has increased 30-fold. While there have been significant advances in all of these areas, a great deal remains to be done. Sickle cell disease is still a major public health problem, and a challenge to the basic scientist, physician, counsellor (and many others) as well as to the community as a whole. Further knowledge should aid in early detection, treatment, and patient care.

The Problem

Medical, psychosocial and socioeconomic problems result from sickle cell disease. All of these deserve attention but only medical problems will be considered in some detail in this monograph.

Most of the important medical problems are the consequences of intravascular sickling, vaso-occlusion and infarction. Small blood vessels supplying various organs and tissues can be partially or completely blocked by sickled erythrocytes (Fig. 3). Such interference with circulation may result in ischemia, pain, necrosis and dysfunction, as well as permanent tissue or organ damage.

Anemia results mainly from the shortened survival time of homozygous S RBC. There are at least two routes for their premature destruction; trauma within the circulation and intravascular hemolysis, or phagocytosis by reticuloendothelial cells in the spleen and liver.

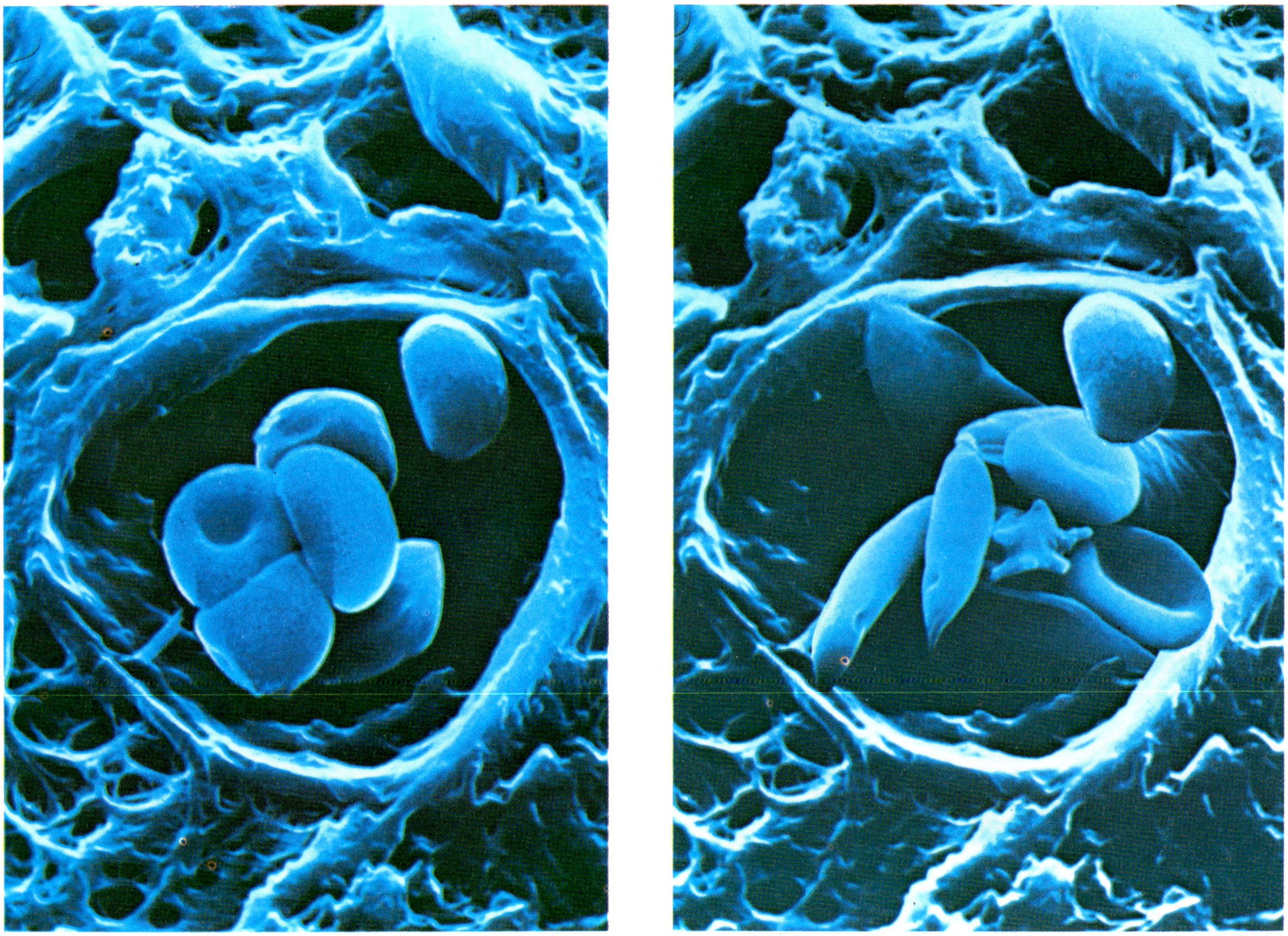

Figure 3. SEM illustrations of blood cell flow in 3-D. **A.** Actual view of flow of normal RBC within a blood vessel (X 9700).

B. A simulation of vaso-occlusion. The sickle cell mass was photographically substituted for the normal RBC seen in A.

The Abnormal Molecule

In sickle cell disease the basic abnormality resides in the globin portion of the hemoglobin molecule. Hemoglobin, the oxygen transporter of the RBC is a conjugate of a pigment, heme, and a protein, globin. The heme component consists of a protoporphyrin in combination with iron in the ferrous state, and accounts for the characteristic red color of hemoglobin. The globin component consists of two pairs of polypeptide chains, with a total of 574 amino acids per hemoglobin molecule. The exact amino acid sequence of each chain has been established.

The major normal adult hemoglobin, designated Hb A, consists of two alpha and two beta chains, ($\alpha_2\beta_2$). Hb A constitutes over 95% of hemoglobin in normal individuals over one year of age, with small amounts (less than 2.5%) of hemoglobins A_2 ($\alpha_2\delta_2$) and F ($\alpha_2\gamma_2$) accounting for the remainder. The exact amino acid sequence for each chain is known.

In some individuals an abnormal Hb results from a genetically determined amino acid substitution in one of the polypeptide chains. The conditions associated with these abnormal hemoglobins are called hemoglobinopathies. Most result from a single amino acid substitution in the β chain, and most are not a disadvantage to the affected individual. One of the exceptions is Hb S, ($\alpha_2\beta_2^S$), as the homozygous state is characterized by significant morbidity. Here the abnormal molecular structure can be directly related to abnormal function and the production of clinical symptoms. Hemoglobin S differs from normal Hb A by one amino acid substitution in the β-chain, namely a valine in place of glutamic acid at the No. 6 position. This substitution on the external surface results in abnormal reactions between molecules of Hb S when oxygen tension is lowered. With deoxygenation the valine substitution permits abnormal polymerization or stacking of Hb S molecules, converting Hb S from the sol to gel state.

Molecular stacking produces stiff rods of Hb S which are the molecular and architectural basis for deforming RBC into rigid, elongated sickle cells (Fig. 4). Ordinary light microscopy revealed these peculiar shaped sickle cells as early as 1910 (Fig. 5).

If an RBC contains predominantly Hb S molecules (as in homozygous S, or S-thalassemia), deoxygenation readily results in polymerization of Hb S molecules and the formation of tactoids with distortion of the cell. However, if RBC contain a significant percentage of another hemoglobin (as A, or F, C, etc.), the dilution effect interferes with molecular stacking as these other hemoglobins have a complementary site for interacting with the valine of Hb S, but have no reactive sites of their own for continuing molecular stacking. Thus heterozygotes (AS) or those with the high F gene in addition to S do not have a great enough concentration of Hb S within RBC to aggregate under normal conditions.

The unusual solubility properties of Hb S provide the basis for the inexpensive screening tests useful in its detection. As will be described later the solubility tests can be modified to differentiate Hb S from other sickling hemoglobins (see p. 76).

Another feature of abnormal hemoglobins is that they frequently have different electrical properties. The laboratory technique of electrophoresis permits separation and identification of molecules on the basis of their surface charge and relative movement in an electric field. More than a hundred different hemoglobin variants have been described. Most of these have been discovered by using electrophoretic techniques. Several relatively simple and inexpensive hemoglobin electrophoresis procedures have been reported. Since electrophoresis can distinguish so many of the hemoglobin variants likely to coexist with Hb S, this test is considered essential for definitive diagnosis of the hemoglobinopathy (see p. 79).

Figure 4. Micrographs to illustrate the distortion of RBC by formation of microcables of Hb S. Interior of RBC is shown in the transmission electron micrograph (X 40000). Note the peripheral ordering of microcables with extension into surface projections. Elsewhere the microcables are sectioned obliquely or in cross-section. Insert is a scanning electron micrograph of the exterior of a different RBC whose interior might be similar to the one shown (X 7700).

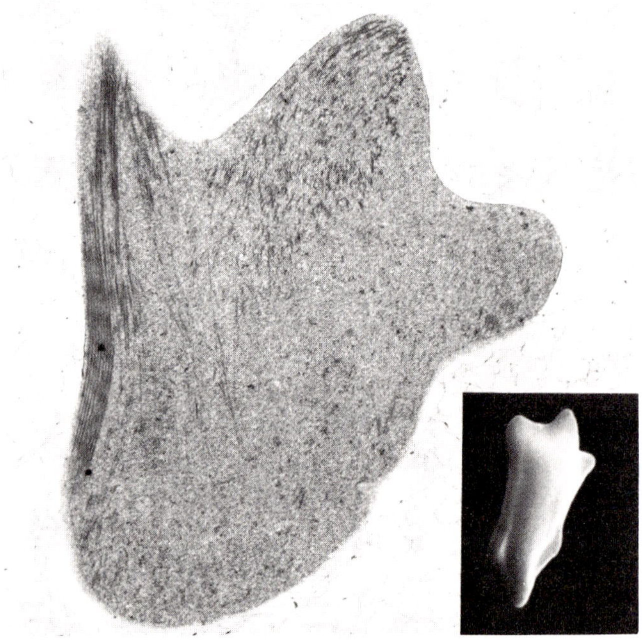

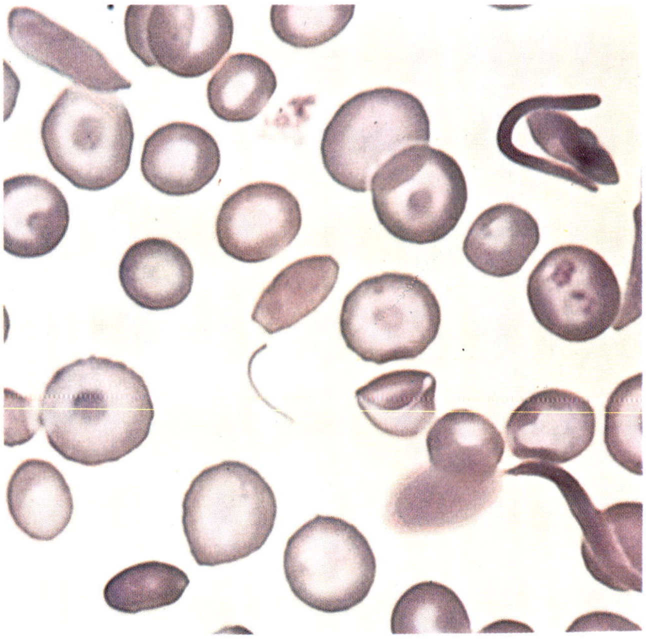

Figure 5. Peripheral blood smear from a Hb SS patient stained with Wright's stain. Note typical sickle cells, target cells, polychromasia.

Hemoglobin Synthesis

Amino acid sequences of specific hemoglobin chains are under genetic control. These chains must then be associated to form tetramer molecules of hemoglobin. Activator genes initiate production of globin chains and repressor genes inhibit the production of globin chains. One operon probably controls the composition and production of each globin chain. The primary structure, presence, absence, or low levels of given globin chains during intrauterine and postnatal life are under control of these genetic mechanisms. Multiple structures and multiple combinations of globin chains are possible. Numerous hemoglobinopathies occur because of these possibilities. The common tetramer types of hemoglobins found in embryonic, fetal and neonatal life are shown in Figure 6. Note that five globin chains are involved ($\alpha, \beta, \gamma, \delta, \epsilon$). The onset, level, and duration of each globin chain is under independent genetic control. Relative production and abundance are shown in Figure 7. The alpha chain appears first, rises to a maximum level, and remains high throughout the life of an individual. Each erythropoietic organ produces α chains (Fig. 8). The epsilon chain normally appears and disappears during the 1st trimester. Comparison of Figures 7 and 8 will infer that the epsilon chain is produced by the yolk sac. In addition, from Figures 6 and 8 one can determine that hemoglobin Gower-2 should be the principle type in the early trimester one period. Hemoglobin Gower-1, a tetramer of epsilon chains probably also appears in this period.

The gamma chain appears during the first trimester, remains at peak levels in trimester two and most of trimester three, and finally falls just prior to parturition, but is still synthesized for several months. Comparison of Figures 6, 7, and 8 indicate that fetal hemoglobin, formed from a dyad of α chains and a dyad of γ chains, is produced primarily by the liver and spleen. Nalbandian, et al, suggested that the peak incidence of abortions near the end of the first trimester may be due to improper genetic switching mechanisms controlling hemoglobin synthesis. Normally, the molecular species of hemoglobin changes from Gower to F during the trimester. These investigators hypothesized that the repressor gene for epsilon chains operates normally but that the activator gene for gamma chains fails to function resulting in non-production of hemoglobin F and a relentless fall in Gower hemoglobin. Anemia and fetal death then

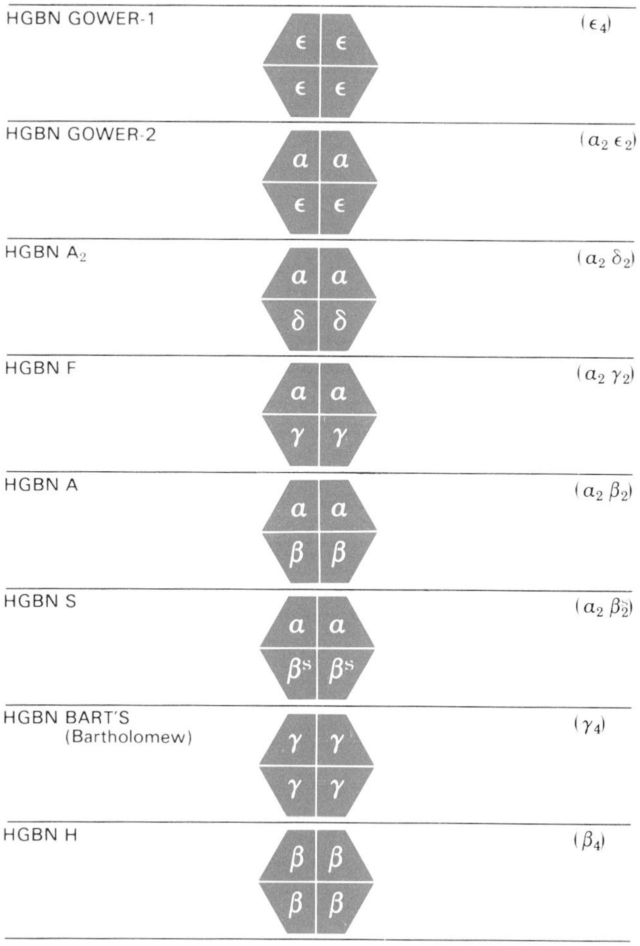

Figure 6. Molecular globin chain combinations found in embryonic, fetal and neonatal life. Each tetramer is formed from dyad associations. Each of the four chains in each molecule is associated with a heme group. The tetramers are named in the left column and conventional notations are given at the right.

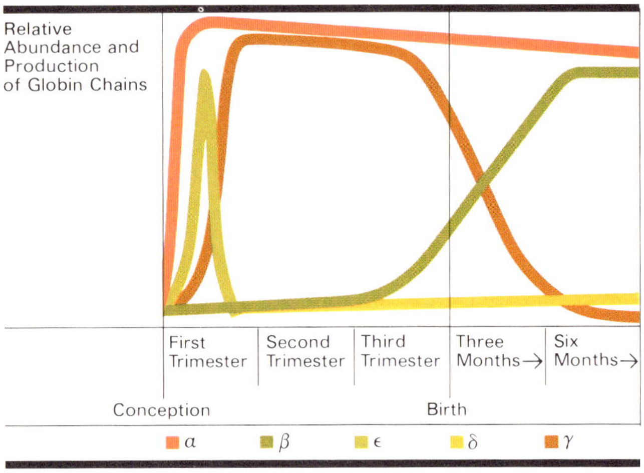

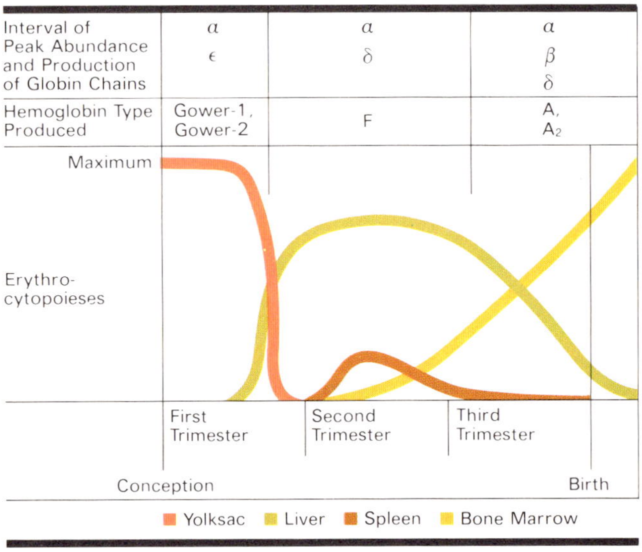

Figure 7. Relative abundance and production of globin chains (alpha, beta, delta, gamma, and epsilon) as a function of intrauterine and neonatal age. Each globin chain associates to form symmetrical dyads which associate with other dyads to form hemoglobin molecules. Tetramer possibilities are given in Figure 6.

Figure 8. Correlation of erythrocytopoiesis in specific organs, peak level of specific globin chains produced, and production of specific hemoglobin types with intrauterine and neonatal life. Compare with Figure 7.

ensue. The peak incidence of fetal death is reported to be later in the trimester than would be expected from these considerations. However, fetal death likely occurs earlier than the actual diagnosis. Fetal age rather than time of abortion should be reported to correlate the incidence of death with changes in genetic control mechanisms.

Referring again to Figures 7 and 8, one can see that as gamma chain production by the liver and spleen diminishes, beta chains are produced principally in the bone marrow by activator genes. There occurs, then, a gradual replacement of fetal hemoglobin by the adult type hemoglobin A. Normally, this conversion is completed by six months after birth. However, persistence of gamma chain production occurs in alpha thalassemia with reduction or absence of alpha chain production. Fetal hemoglobin may then persist well into adult life. Tetramers of gamma globin chains may also occur as hemoglobin Bart's (see Figures 6 and 7) and may account for sickling at birth. In time hemoglobin Bart's may be replaced by hemoglobin H, a tetramer of beta chains. Coexistence of hemoglobin Bart's and H have been reported in alpha thalassemia. Presumably the repressor gene for gamma chains fails to act while the activator gene for beta chains operates normally, all while alpha chains are reduced or absent. It is also possible that there is a decrease or defect in messenger RNA that could affect alpha chain synthesis. In any case, in beta thalassemia the production of beta chains is reduced or absent and it can be expected that hemoglobin F will persist as well as the appearance of hemoglobin A_2, a tetramer of alpha and delta chains. Rare hemoglobinopathies such as tetramers of alpha chains, delta chains, and beta chains can be accounted for on the basis of genetic controlling mechanisms.

Sickle cell hemoglobin results from a genetic substitution of valine for glutamic acid in the 6th position from the N-terminal end of beta chains. Production of this abnormal hemoglobin would not be expected before the later stages of trimester three when beta chains begin to be produced by the bone marrow (Figs. 6, 7 and 8). Even at birth, levels of sickle cell hemoglobin, either in the homozygous (SS) or heterozygous (AS) states, may be too low for detection by sickling or solubility tests. Screening in the neonate, for this reason, should not be attempted with sickling or solubility tests. Note also from Figure 8 that, when sickle cell hemoglobin occurs in the homozygous state (SS), sickling crises usually would not be expected prior to 3 months after birth until the abnormal hemoglobin reaches higher levels in relation to the levels of hemoglobin F. It is clear that hemoglobin F affords protection against sickling by Hb S.

The Erythrocyte

Normal RBC are membrane limited objects filled with hemoglobin in a soluble and relatively fluid state. When viewed in 3-dimensional relief most RBC (93 ± 5%) are smooth surfaced and exist as biconcave discs which are very flexible (Fig. 9). A continual surface shimmering effect is noticeable from the disc forms of living RBC. This surface flicker is one sign of the extreme plasticity of normal RBC. Alterations in shape tend to decrease this plasticity so essential for normal flow within the fine caliber vessels of the microcirculation.

In sickle cell disease the RBC have the capability of drastic shape change and loss of flexibility because of their hemoglobin S content. RBC from individuals with sickle cell anemia contain from 80-100% hemoglobin S. Sickle cell trait subjects are fairly resistant to sickling stimuli because their RBC contain only 20-45% hemoglobin S.

Situations of low O_2 tension, acidosis and dehydration can promote the peculiar elongated or crescent shaped sickle cells (Fig. 10). Sickling stimuli may occur locally (as in a single vessel or organ) or may be more generalized (as in the case of generalized hypoxia during anesthesia). As there is physiologic variation in levels of tissue oxygenation and acidity, certain organs pose more hazard to circulatory flow of hemoglobin S containing erythrocytes (Fig. 11). Examples are organs (spleen, liver, renal medulla) where blood flow is slow and organs (brain, muscle, maternal placenta) where the high metabolic rate extracts more oxygen from the blood.

For a time sickle shape changes are reversible. Several sickle-desickle transitions or extreme sickling may injure the RBC irreparably. Such cells are termed irreversible sickle cells and are quite rigid (Fig. 12). Dependent upon the magnitude of the injury, a sickled cell has several options. It may reverse to its former relatively normal biconcave

9

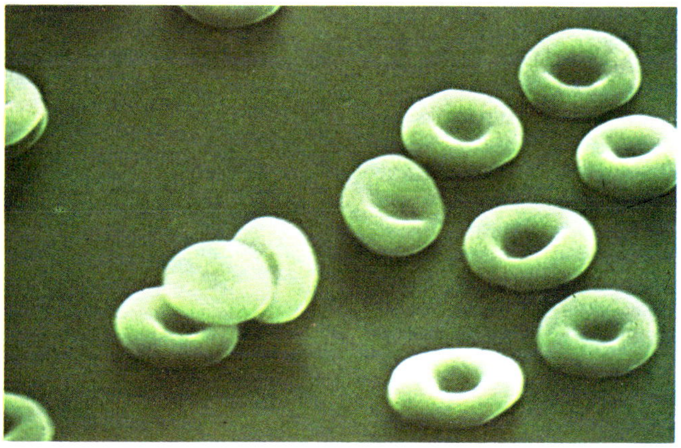

10

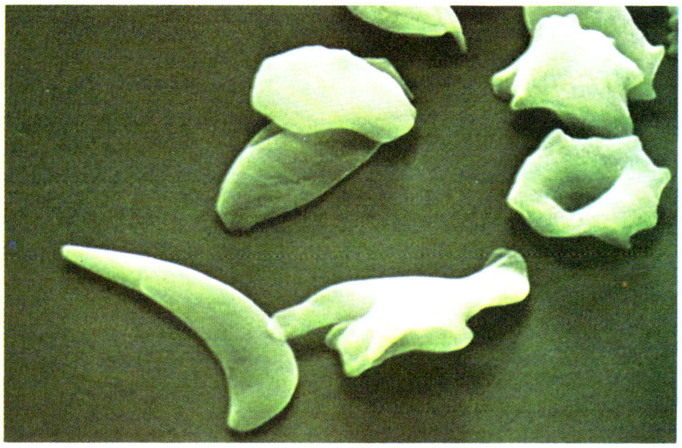

11

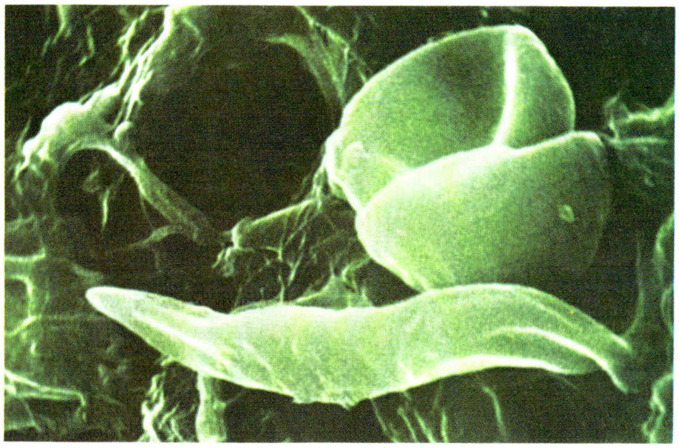

Figure 9. Normal RBC from Hb AA subject as seen in 3-D by SEM (X 5230).
Figure 10. Sickled RBC from Hb SS subject viewed by SEM. These RBC appear to be rigid (X 7100).
Figure 11. SEM of a surgically removed spleen from a Hb SS patient. The sickle cell and 2 rather normal appearing RBC are in the splenic cord area of the red pulp (X 22300).

Figure 15. Various forms of RBC seen with Nomarski optics. In differential counts these cell shapes are identified and counted. **A.** Biconcave discs with a small flat platelet disc at the left. **B.** A target cell in the center flanked by biconcave discs. **C.** Crenated forms. Two crenated discs (scallops) and three crenated sphere (burrs) are in the field. **D.** Note flat disc at bottom right near biconcave discs. **E.** Spherocyte (upper) and spiny sphere (lower). **F.** Mostly spherocytes. **G.** Hemolysis finger type at far right. **H.** Two RBC ghosts (membranes after release of hemoglobin by osmotic hemolysis) are located centrally in field of spherocytes (SEM X 2200).

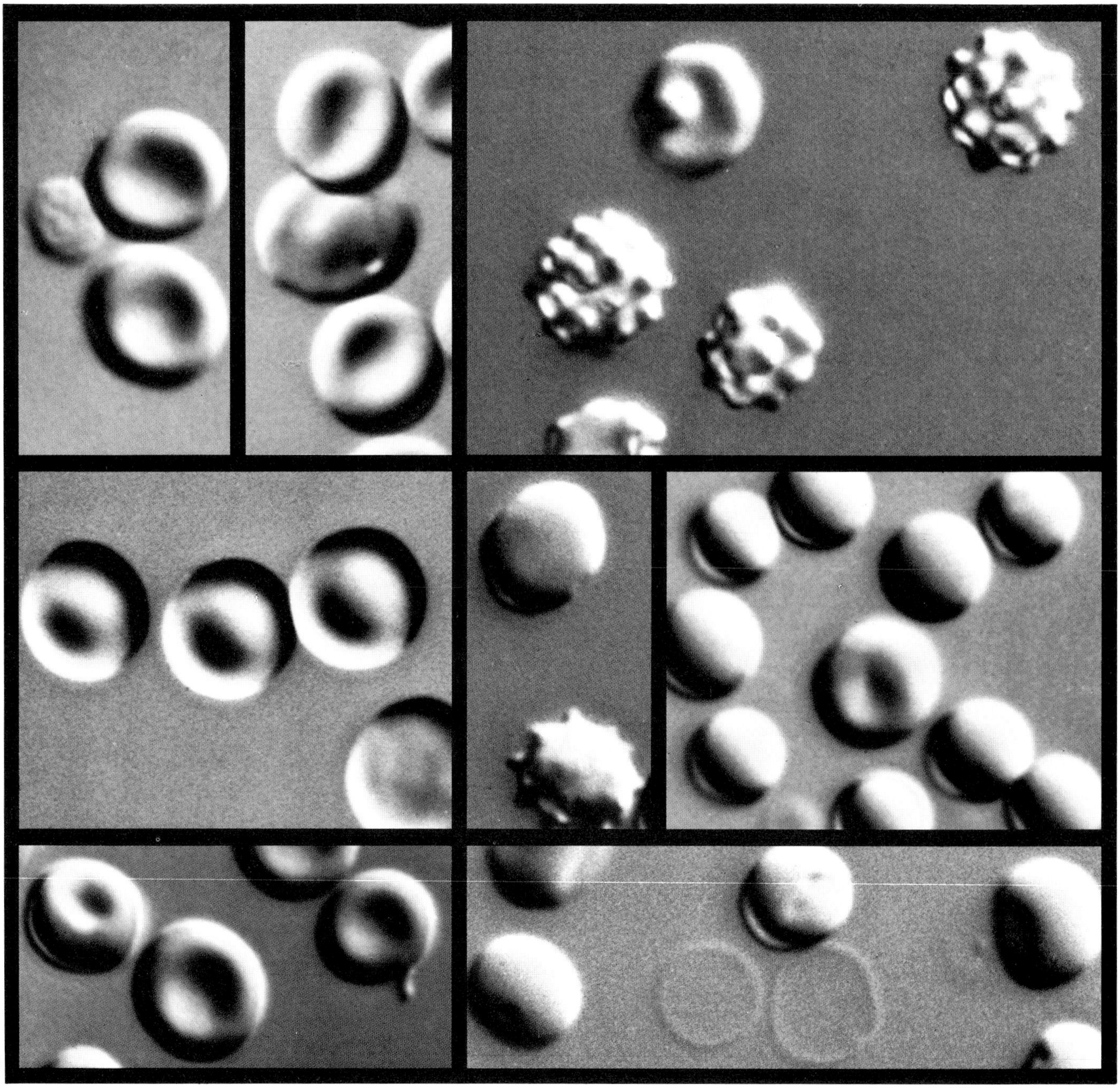

A B C

D E F

G H

The Erythrocyte

Normal RBC are membrane limited objects filled with hemoglobin in a soluble and relatively fluid state. When viewed in 3-dimensional relief most RBC (93 ± 5%) are smooth surfaced and exist as biconcave discs which are very flexible (Fig. 9). A continual surface shimmering effect is noticeable from the disc forms of living RBC. This surface flicker is one sign of the extreme plasticity of normal RBC. Alterations in shape tend to decrease this plasticity so essential for normal flow within the fine caliber vessels of the microcirculation.

In sickle cell disease the RBC have the capability of drastic shape change and loss of flexibility because of their hemoglobin S content. RBC from individuals with sickle cell anemia contain from 80-100% hemoglobin S. Sickle cell trait subjects are fairly resistant to sickling stimuli because their RBC contain only 20-45% hemoglobin S.

Situations of low O_2 tension, acidosis and dehydration can promote the peculiar elongated or crescent shaped sickle cells (Fig. 10). Sickling stimuli may occur locally (as in a single vessel or organ) or may be more generalized (as in the case of generalized hypoxia during anesthesia). As there is physiologic variation in levels of tissue oxygenation and acidity, certain organs pose more hazard to circulatory flow of hemoglobin S containing erythrocytes (Fig. 11). Examples are organs (spleen, liver, renal medulla) where blood flow is slow and organs (brain, muscle, maternal placenta) where the high metabolic rate extracts more oxygen from the blood.

For a time sickle shape changes are reversible. Several sickle-desickle transitions or extreme sickling may injure the RBC irreparably. Such cells are termed irreversible sickle cells and are quite rigid (Fig. 12). Dependent upon the magnitude of the injury, a sickled cell has several options. It may reverse to its former relatively normal biconcave

9

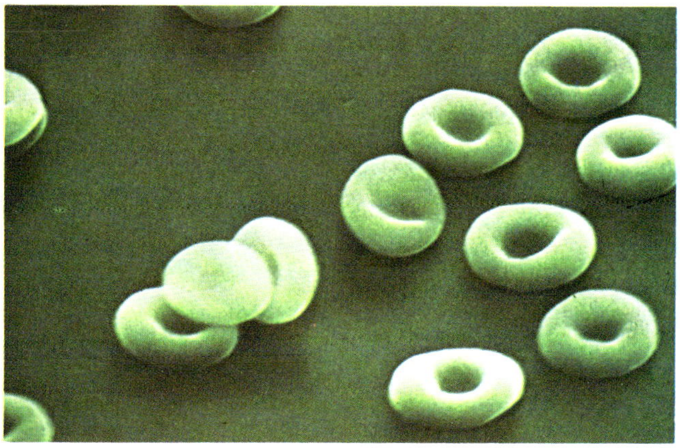

10

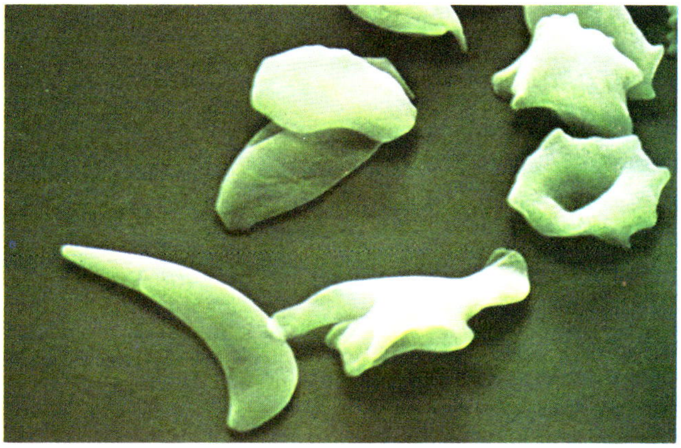

11

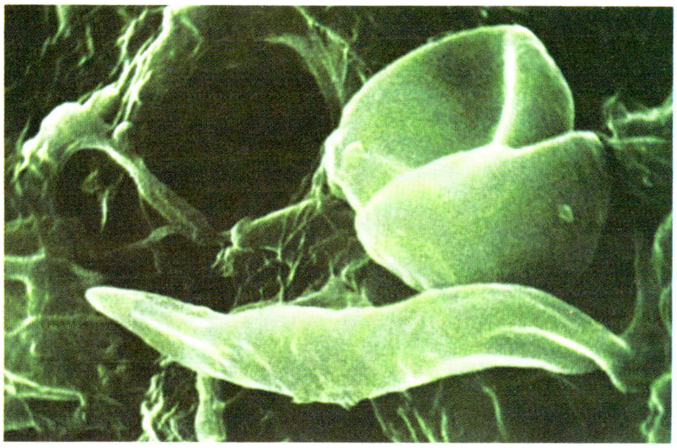

Figure 9. Normal RBC from Hb AA subject as seen in 3-D by SEM (X 5230).
Figure 10. Sickled RBC from Hb SS subject viewed by SEM. These RBC appear to be rigid (X 7100).
Figure 11. SEM of a surgically removed spleen from a Hb SS patient. The sickle cell and 2 rather normal appearing RBC are in the splenic cord area of the red pulp (X 22300).

Figure 15. Various forms of RBC seen with Nomarski optics. In differential counts these cell shapes are identified and counted. **A.** Biconcave discs with a small flat platelet disc at the left. **B.** A target cell in the center flanked by biconcave discs. **C.** Crenated forms. Two crenated discs (scallops) and three crenated sphere (burrs) are in the field. **D.** Note flat disc at bottom right near biconcave discs. **E.** Spherocyte (upper) and spiny sphere (lower). **F.** Mostly spherocytes. **G.** Hemolysis finger type at far right. **H.** Two RBC ghosts (membranes after release of hemoglobin by osmotic hemolysis) are located centrally in field of spherocytes (SEM X 2200).

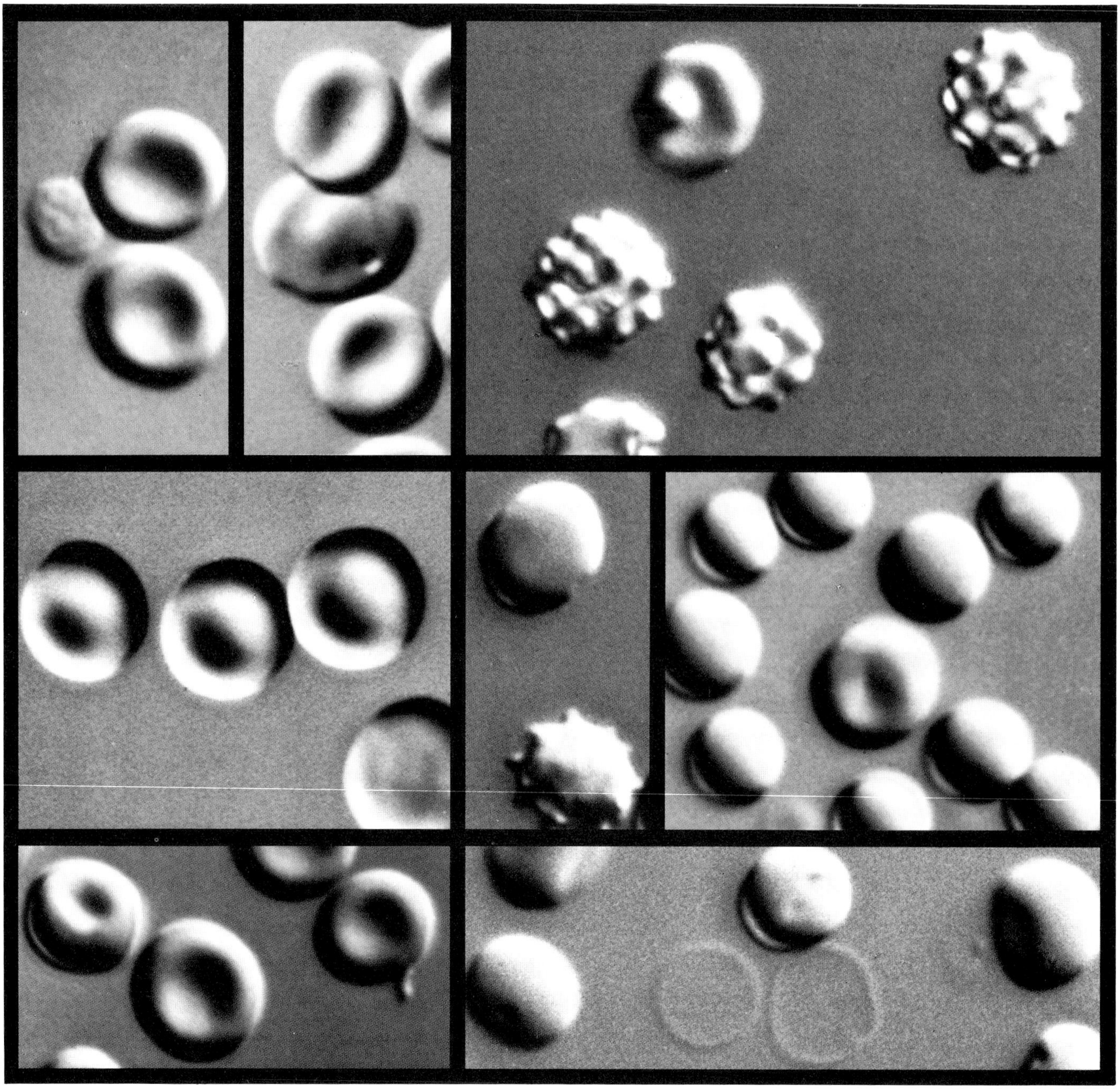

A B C

D E F

G H

The Erythrocyte

Normal RBC are membrane limited objects filled with hemoglobin in a soluble and relatively fluid state. When viewed in 3-dimensional relief most RBC (93 $\pm$ 5%) are smooth surfaced and exist as biconcave discs which are very flexible (Fig. 9). A continual surface shimmering effect is noticeable from the disc forms of living RBC. This surface flicker is one sign of the extreme plasticity of normal RBC. Alterations in shape tend to decrease this plasticity so essential for normal flow within the fine caliber vessels of the microcirculation.

In sickle cell disease the RBC have the capability of drastic shape change and loss of flexibility because of their hemoglobin S content. RBC from individuals with sickle cell anemia contain from 80-100% hemoglobin S. Sickle cell trait subjects are fairly resistant to sickling stimuli because their RBC contain only 20-45% hemoglobin S.

Situations of low O_2 tension, acidosis and dehydration can promote the peculiar elongated or crescent shaped sickle cells (Fig. 10). Sickling stimuli may occur locally (as in a single vessel or organ) or may be more generalized (as in the case of generalized hypoxia during anesthesia). As there is physiologic variation in levels of tissue oxygenation and acidity, certain organs pose more hazard to circulatory flow of hemoglobin S containing erythrocytes (Fig. 11). Examples are organs (spleen, liver, renal medulla) where blood flow is slow and organs (brain, muscle, maternal placenta) where the high metabolic rate extracts more oxygen from the blood.

For a time sickle shape changes are reversible. Several sickle-desickle transitions or extreme sickling may injure the RBC irreparably. Such cells are termed irreversible sickle cells and are quite rigid (Fig. 12). Dependent upon the magnitude of the injury, a sickled cell has several options. It may reverse to its former relatively normal biconcave

9

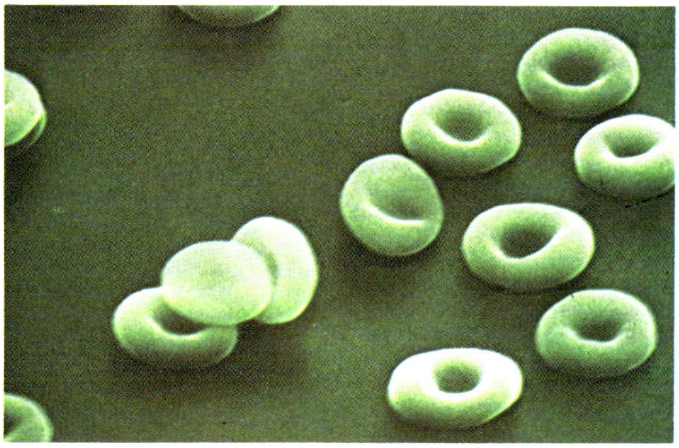

10

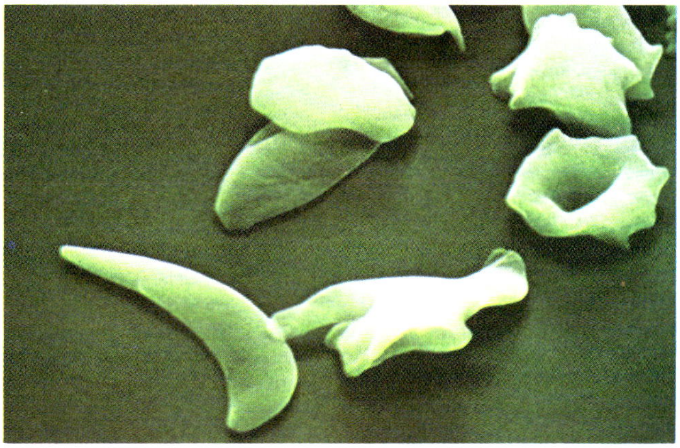

11

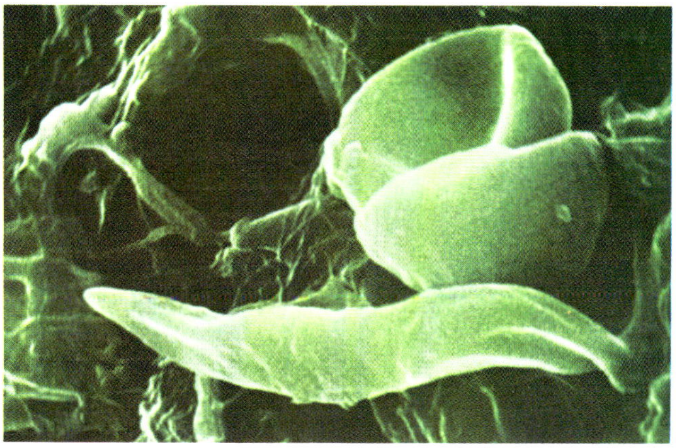

Figure 9. Normal RBC from Hb AA subject as seen in 3-D by SEM (X 5230).
Figure 10. Sickled RBC from Hb SS subject viewed by SEM. These RBC appear to be rigid (X 7100).
Figure 11. SEM of a surgically removed spleen from a Hb SS patient. The sickle cell and 2 rather normal appearing RBC are in the splenic cord area of the red pulp (X 22300).

12

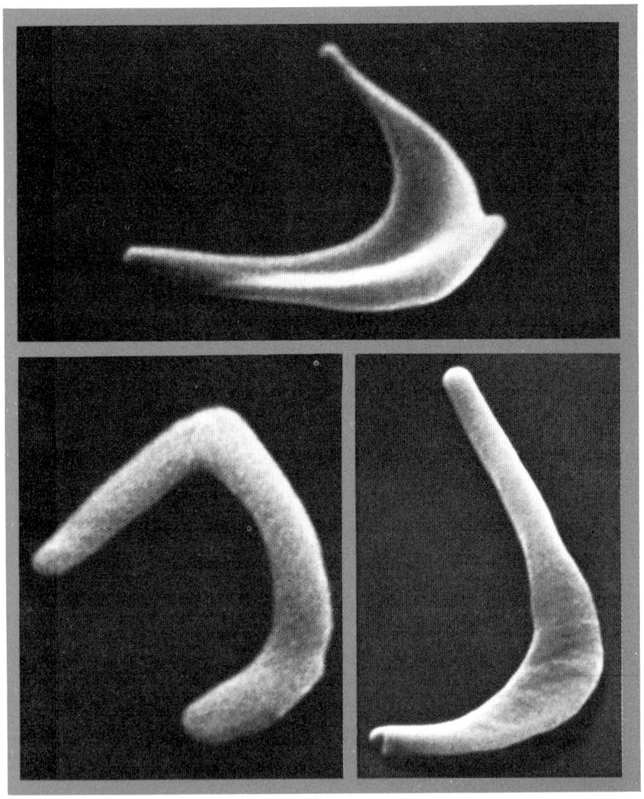

13

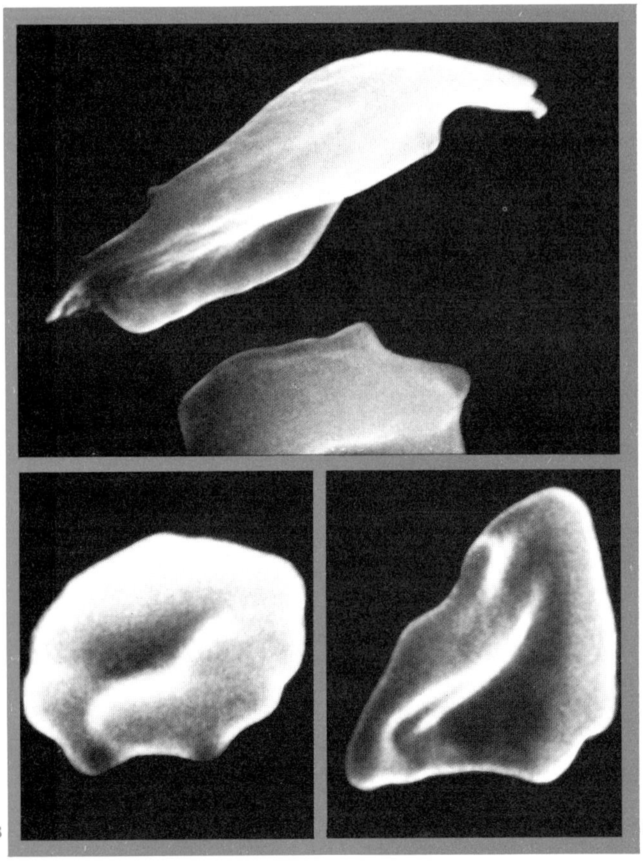

Figure 12. Some examples of irreversibly sickled RBC by SEM (X 7800).
Figure 13. A SEM composite simulates a possible desickling sequence (A-C). Note surface ridging in lower projection of stage 1 which may reflect underlying microcables of Hb S. Most likely stage 4 would be a symmetrical binconcave disc (X 8000).

disc form retaining a degree of flexibility (Fig. 13) or it may hemolyze and be prematurely destroyed. Of greatest significance, sickled cells may intertwine and form relatively rigid masses that block blood flow to tissues or organs. Transient or permanent injury may result as local circulatory flow is compromised by these sickle cell "log jams" as shown in Fig. 3.

THE REWARDS OF MICROSCOPY

A variety of microscopy techniques (light and electron microscopy as well as cinemicrography) have provided valuable visual clues regarding the phenomena of sickling and have rewarded investigators concerned with the fundamental basis of the disease. Certain questions can be answered best by applied microscopy. This section will consider three sets of questions concerned with (1) morphology and physiology of sickling, (2) quantitative RBC microscopy and (3) ultrastructure of sickling.

Greatest appreciation of this section is gained if the reader recognizes that microscopy as other technology requires understanding of its advantages and limitations. Only then and with strict controls can microscopy be applied to yield data that is instructive and has utility.

Some Technical Detail Important for Microscopy Selection and Data Interpretation

Objectives must be clearly defined. The interest may be to identify sickle cells *ex vivo*. The goal may be to examine the sickling-desickling cycle in action using cinemicrography. If one desires information on the status of RBC shape within the circulation, fixation must be immediate on exit of blood from the puncture site. Temporary venous stasis, induced by tourniquet preparatory to sampling, induces a varying degree of deoxygenation. To minimize this, a tourniquet should not be used, or if used, should be released as soon as the needle is in the vein. The first relatively stagnant blood drawn should be discarded and only the rapid flow used.

Optical Systems. Stained cells are best viewed with ordinary optics. Unstained cells, living or fixed, are best observed with Nomarski optics (combination of contrast interference and phase optics) attached to the light microscope. Although phase optics alone can be instructive there is greater distortion of cell shape. With the Nomarski system images appear in 3-dimensional form. This system has particular value when quantitation of cells is attempted in terms of their shape. Moreover, application of cinemicrography permits striking visual displays of living cells "in action" (Fig. 14).

Types of RBC Preparations. Two kinds of cell preparations are particularly suitable for light microscopic study. By far the most often used in hospitals and clinics are *peripheral blood smears* stained with one of the Romanowsky stains (Leishman's, Wright's, etc.). Peripheral smears consist of cells variably flattened and distorted in the preparation process but show rather well the extreme sickle forms in homozygous S disease (Fig. 5). (In contrast sickle forms are almost never encountered in peripheral blood smears from AS subjects.)

Wet mount preparations are even better for microscopy as the fluid environment protects the cells. Stains are unnecessary. When venous blood samples have been properly collected and anticoagulated (3.2% sodium citrate or heparin), RBC shape observed in wet mounts is more likely reflective of that *in vivo*. Also one can see various stages in the sickling process, and can observe living cells in motion and actually "stop action" when desired by killing with a fixative. For minimizing artifacts, buffered glutaraldehyde proved superior to formalin fixation.

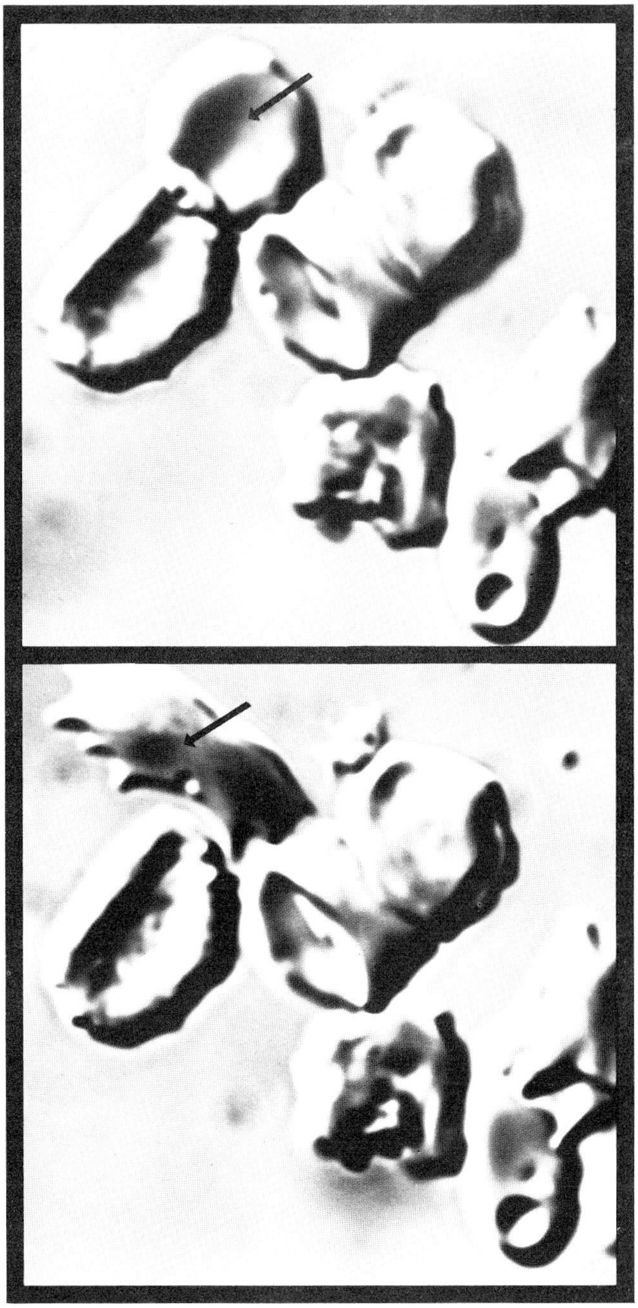

Figure 14. Sickling in action (arrow) taken from a film sequence of effect of oxygen deprivation on Hb SS erythrocytes (X 2330).

Figure 15. Various forms of RBC seen with Nomarski optics. In differential counts these cell shapes are identified and counted. **A.** Biconcave discs with a small flat platelet disc at the left. **B.** A target cell in the center flanked by biconcave discs. **C.** Crenated forms. Two crenated discs (scallops) and three crenated sphere (burrs) are in the field. **D.** Note flat disc at bottom right near biconcave discs. **E.** Spherocyte (upper) and spiny sphere (lower). **F.** Mostly spherocytes. **G.** Hemolysis finger type at far right. **H.** Two RBC ghosts (membranes after release of hemoglobin by osmotic hemolysis) are located centrally in field of spherocytes (SEM X 2200).

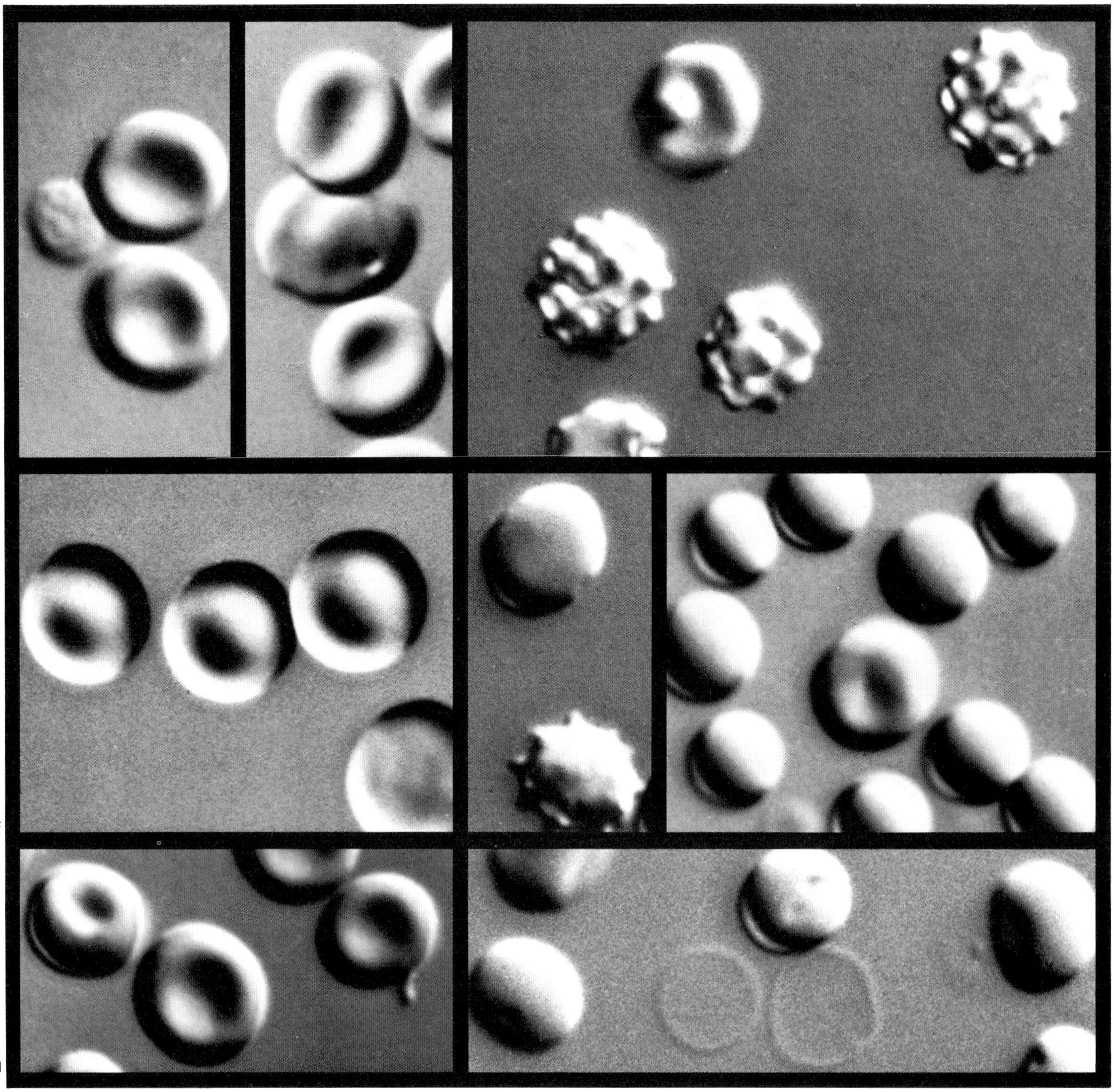

A B C

D E F

G H

RBC Differential Counts. Our standard laboratory procedure utilizes fresh, non-stagnant, anticoagulated and fixed blood in sealed wet mounts. Viewing and photography employ a Nomarski optical system. RBC appear as 3-dimensional images (Fig. 15). It is relatively easy to count 500 cells, classifying them on the basis of their 3-D shape. These classes are biconcave discs, flat discs, spherocytes, crenated discs (scalloped edged), crenated spheres (burr and spiny forms), and sickle cells (holly leafs, crescents, cigars and oat seed forms).

Morphology and Physiology of Sickling

The first set of questions considers the appearance and reactivity of RBC containing hemoglobin S. What does a sickle cell look like, and are these cells pathognomonic of sickle cell anemia? Are there certain anatomic sites where sickle stimuli are more profound? Do all RBC containing Hb S have the same sensitivity to sickling stimuli?

As early as 1910, Herrick, using ordinary light microscopy, reported his observations of strange sickle shaped RBC in the peripheral blood smear of a black West Indian student. Optical systems have improved greatly since Herrick's time, and light microscopy still offers considerable practical value for detection of sickle cells (as well as evaluation of blood cell morphology in general). For many years such a visual demonstration was considered diagnostic of sickle cell anemia (Fig. 5). We now know that it is only presumptive evidence of sickle cell anemia, particularly if the hemoglobin value is between 6 and 8 gms %. However, the definitive diagnosis of sickle cell anemia requires additional knowledge of hemoglobin solubility and electrophoretic behavior.

Significant information can also be gained by inducing sickling *ex vivo* (Fig. 15). This may occur spontaneously as cells use up their available O_2 resources in sealed wet mount preparations or test tubes, or oxygen tension can be lowered by incubating the cells in the presence of sodium metabisulfite, a reducing agent. (The latter provides the basis for a widely used screening test, the "sickle cell prep." See p. 76.) For experimental work, more exact levels of deoxygenation can be achieved by equilibrating blood with specific gas mixtures of oxygen and nitrogen.

Data from rigidly controlled and standardized testing permit the following conclusions. The magnitude of sickling is greater in Hb SS than sickle trait subjects. The extent of sickling, however, varies among individuals with Hb SS. The rate and extent of sickling are not uniform within a given RBC population. Some cells sickle in seconds while others resist and show fairly normal morphology for hours. Probably the past history of the individual cells conditions their response to sickle stressors. Certainly their content of Hb F, which is distributed heterogeneously among homozygous S RBC, is another factor (Fig. 16). Also quite important is the actual oxygen tension of the fluid environment. Even normal flexible RBC are stiffened at $PO_2 < 30$ mm Hg. Thus vascular beds in organs such as spleen and maternal placenta provide an environment most conducive to sickling.

Quantitative Microscopy

The second group of questions to be answered concern the feasibility and benefits to be gained from quantitative microscopy. Why perform RBC differential counts? Can such differential counts be of benefit in assessing a patient's status, or in clinical trials to evaluate the effectiveness of an investigational agent?

Quantitation of the sickling response or other RBC pathophysiology is possible, but has been primarily a research tool to date, being done only in a few specialized centers. For reproducibility and reliability

Figure 16. Various sickle forms seen with Nomarski optics. **A-E.** Extreme sickle forms, i.e. oat seed in A, banana or cigar shape in D. **F-J.** Holly leaf forms, some spread, rough surfaced. **K.** Some early sickle forms with Hb margination and widening of central concavity (SEM X 2200).

A B C D E

F G H

I J K

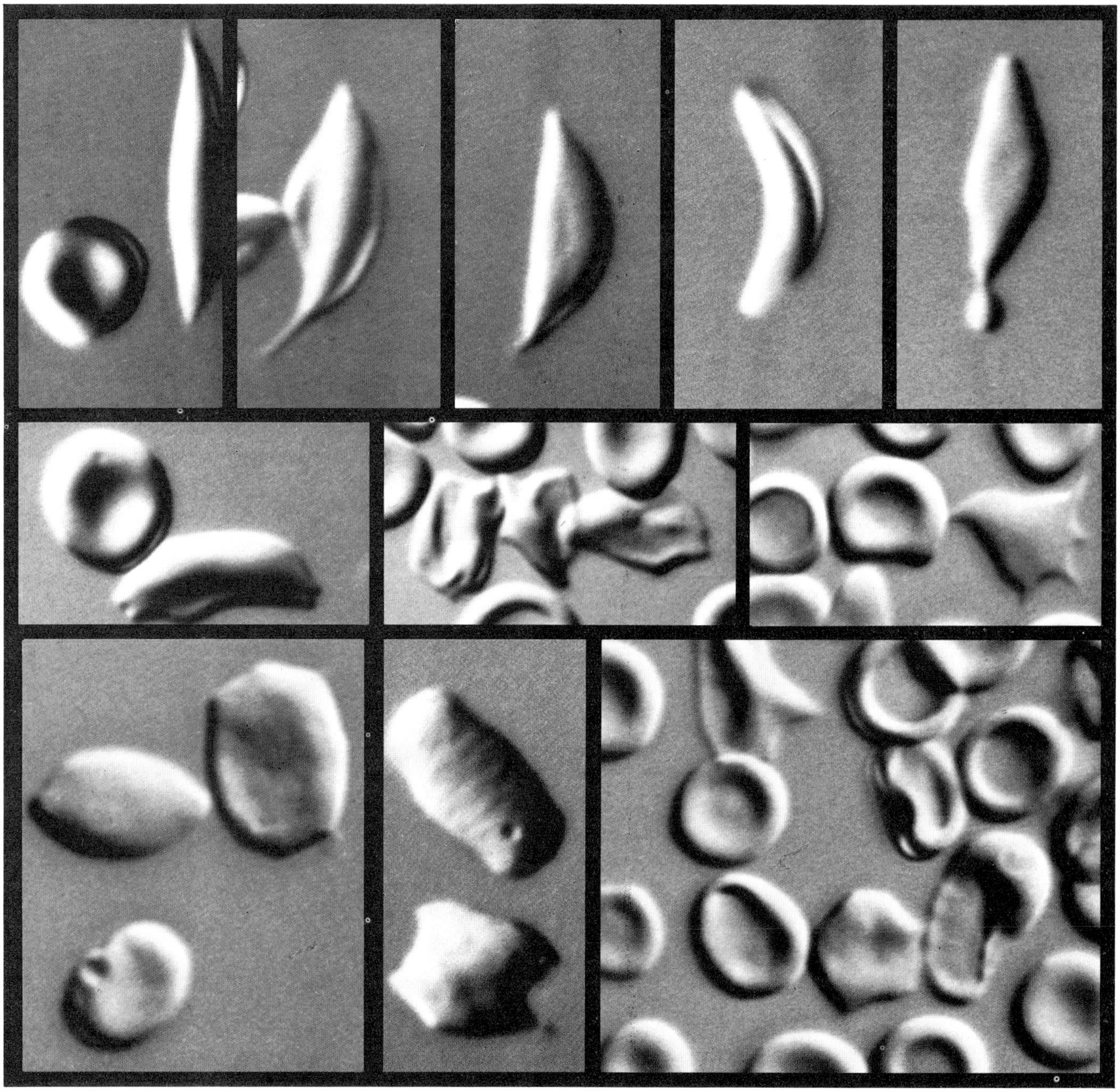

clearly defined conditions and concurrent controls are necessary. If these conditions are met, results can offer an objective gauge of RBC status. On the basis of the 3-dimensional shapes of RBC it is easily possible to classify them into groups that have certain functional implications.

Frequently the RBC form is reflective of the functional state of the cell. Normal RBC exist predominantly as biconcave discs (93.2 ± 5.1%) which are partially collapsed spheres of great flexibility (Fig. 15). Faulty water and salt control can produce swelling, first appearing as flat discs and later as spherocytes (Fig. 17). When ATP energy is depleted or when RBC are in a hypertonic environment, crenated cells result (Fig. 17). Sickle cells and target cells illustrate internal polymerization of Hb S or crystallization of Hb C, resulting in reduced flexibility (Fig. 18). Schistocytes or fragmented forms are the remains of grossly damaged RBC (Fig. 19). The percentage of these and other RBC forms may illustrate the type and magnitude of the hematologic insult (Table A).

Although used to date only as a research tool, quantitative data such as described may be instructive in patient management or aid evaluation of drug activity. Comparison of sequential samples taken at intervals during a clinical episode will no doubt be more instructive than single specimens. In our experience such cell quantitation does not always parallel the clinical evaluation of severity. However, it is important to consider that *in vivo* sickling and vascular obstruction in certain areas may be clinically silent, yet significant as some degree of permanent injury may be occurring. Also, sequential sample analysis or concurrent comparative work on a single specimen shows promise as an objective gauge of drug efficacy. Hopefully progress and interest in this area of investigation will continue.

Figure 17. Distribution of fetal hemoglobin by the acid elution technique. **A.** Note heterogeneous pattern in sickle cell anemia. **B.** Cord blood sample for comparison. **C.** Normal adult cells appear as ghosts by this method.

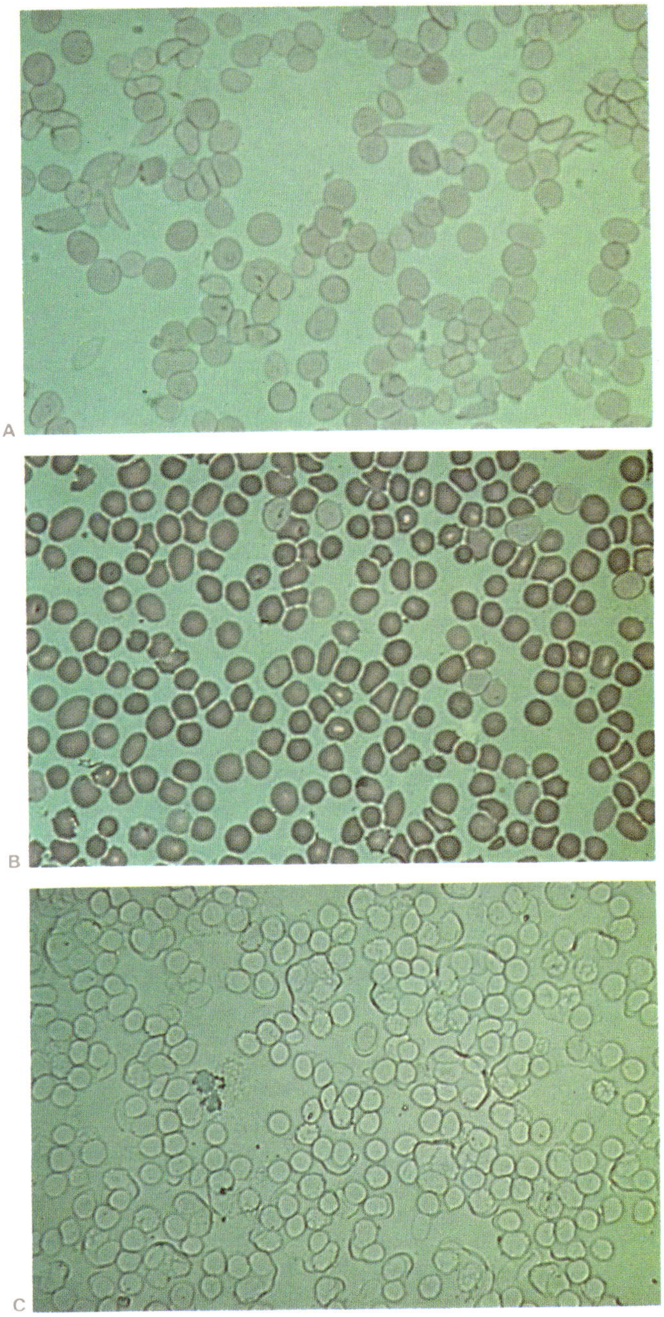
A
B
C

Figure 18. Various RBC forms that most likely would exhibit reduced flexibility. **A.** Irregular spherocyte. Note pitting which probably occurred in the spleen. **B.** Crenated discs and spheres (burrs). **C.** Sickle cells, target cell and hemolyzing or vesiculating RBC. **D.** Hb C crystal in RBC. Also note various degrees of swelling and a microspherocyte (SEM X 2200).

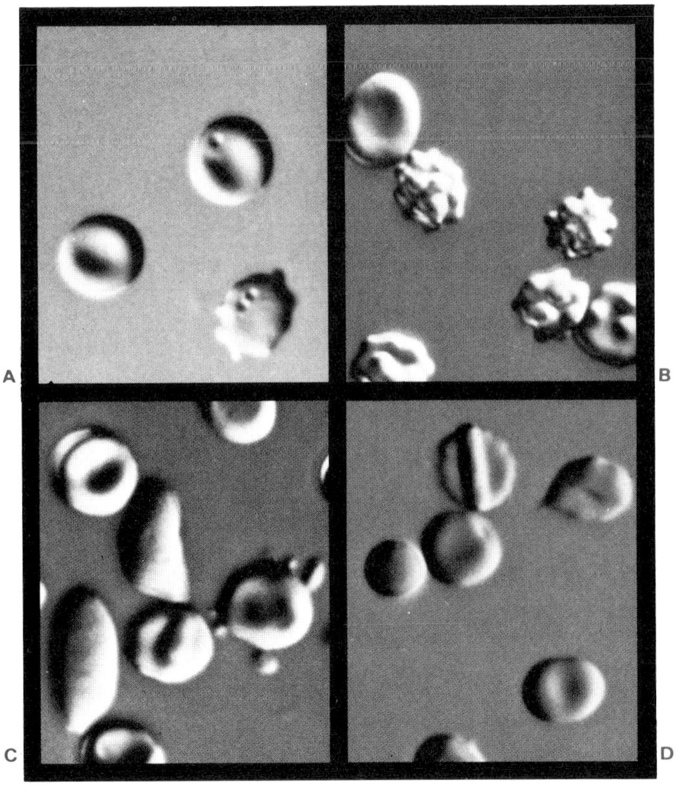

Figure 19. Schistocytes (RBC fragments) of various shapes are seen by SEM (X 2200). Compare size and shape of schistocytes with the normal biconcave discs seen in fields A-F. Membrane shedding or vesiculation appears centrally in field A. The microbiconcave disc seen centrally in field D might originate by further membrane loss from schistocytes seen in field G; note membrane loss, also, may produce a microspherocyte.

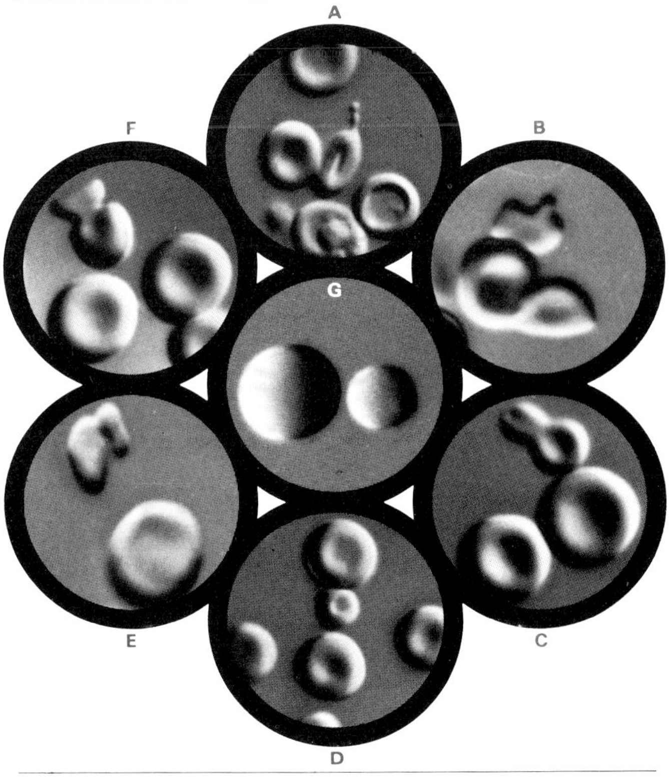

Table A
Quantitative microscopy illustrating *ex vivo* effects of either sodium metabisulfite or hypertonic sodium chloride on selected hemoglobinopathies

Experiment		Percent Erythrocyte Types (Nomarski Images) Biconcave discs	Crenated forms	Sickle forms	Crystal containing	Schistocytes	Other* forms
1. Fixation Immediate							
	Hb AA	97	0	0	0	1	2
	Hb SS	60	0	36	0	1	3
	Hb CC	82	0	0	0	9	9
2. Plus PBS**							
	Hb AA	94	3	0	0	1	2
3. Plus $Na_2S_2O_5$***							
	Hb AA	42	54	0	0	1	3
	Hb SS	22	0	76	0	1	1
4. Plus NaCl****							
	Hb AA	52	37	0	0	1	10
	Hb SS	44	22	27		1	6
	Hb CC	29	7	0	54	2	8

These citrate anticoagulated blood specimens were fixed in buffered glutaraldehyde either immediately or at end of incubation period with test reagent.

* Flat discs, spherocytes or bizarre shapes.
** Potassium phosphate buffered saline pH 7.4; fluid concentration 0.9%
*** Sodium metabisulfite; final concentration 1%, 15 min. incubation.
**** Potassium phosphate buffered saline, pH 7.4; final concentration 1.5%, incubation 3 hr.

Ultrastructure of Sickling

The third set of questions concern the fine structural changes that result as cells sickle. Is there a visible change within the cell interior? What happens to Hb S on deoxygenation? Does sickling produce membrane injury? Is there a fixed pattern of RBC deformation during the sickle-desickle transition?

Transition from a normal appearing biconcave disc to an obvious sickle form occurs rapidly (10-15 sec.) in the most sensitive cells (Fig. 20). A few cells resist sickling stimuli for hours.

Several patterns of sickling can be seen when the phenemona are observed in action under Nomarski or phase optics. One visual event, loss of surface flicker or shimmering, is common to development of the various bizarre forms (poikilocytes). The ultimate shape assumed relates to the cell's past history, present biochemistry and the magnitude of oxygen deficiency.

While RBC can engage in several sickle-desickle cycles with a return to near normal shape and flexibility, sickling can produce serious membrane injury. A severe injury may permanently stiffen or deform, even at usually adequate oxygen pressures. Signs of membrane injury and/or loss are especially evident with the aid of 3-D microscopy (Fig. 21). Repeatedly sickled cells frequently exhibit rough textured or wrinkled surfaces in contrast to the fine textured smooth surface of normal cells (Fig. 22). Some of the roughened patches may be injured membrane associated with irreversibly denatured Hb S. Freeze cleavage technique plus transmission electron microscopy show the internal membrane of irreversibly sickled cells to have occasional tiny tufts which may represent denatured Hb S bound to the membrane.

Membrane and hemoglobin loss may show up as surface pits or scars even with the Nomarski type

Figure 20. A simulation of sickling derived from SEM. Note elongation of RBC, margination of Hb and stiffening of RBC in right panel (X 7800).

20

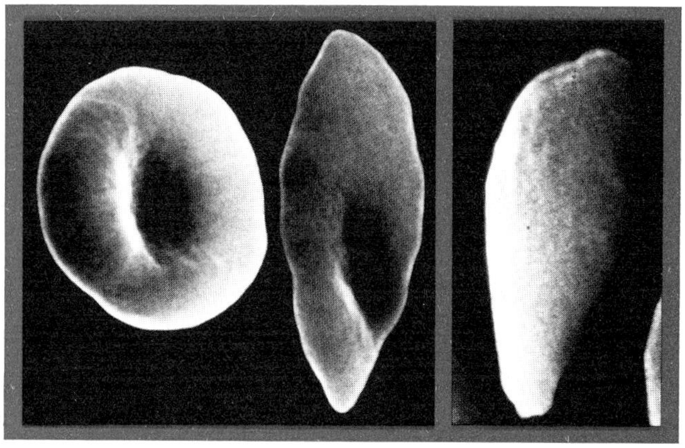

21

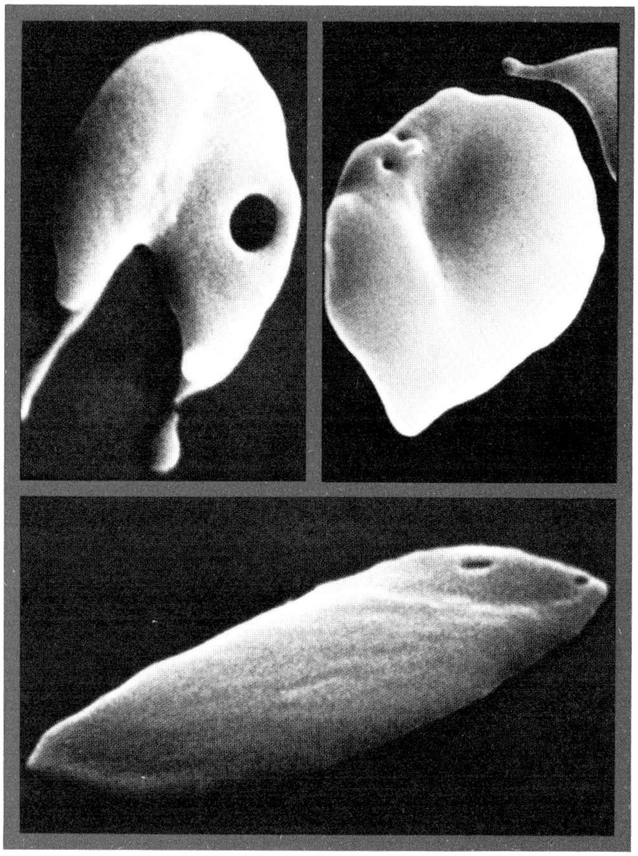

Figure 21. Signs of membrane injury (holes or pits) in several sickle cells viewed by SEM (X 8400).

Figure 22. Membrane roughness is featured in some of these deoxygenated RBC seen by SEM. Observe that 2 of these are biconcave discs. The apparent rigidity of these RBC is notable (X 12000).

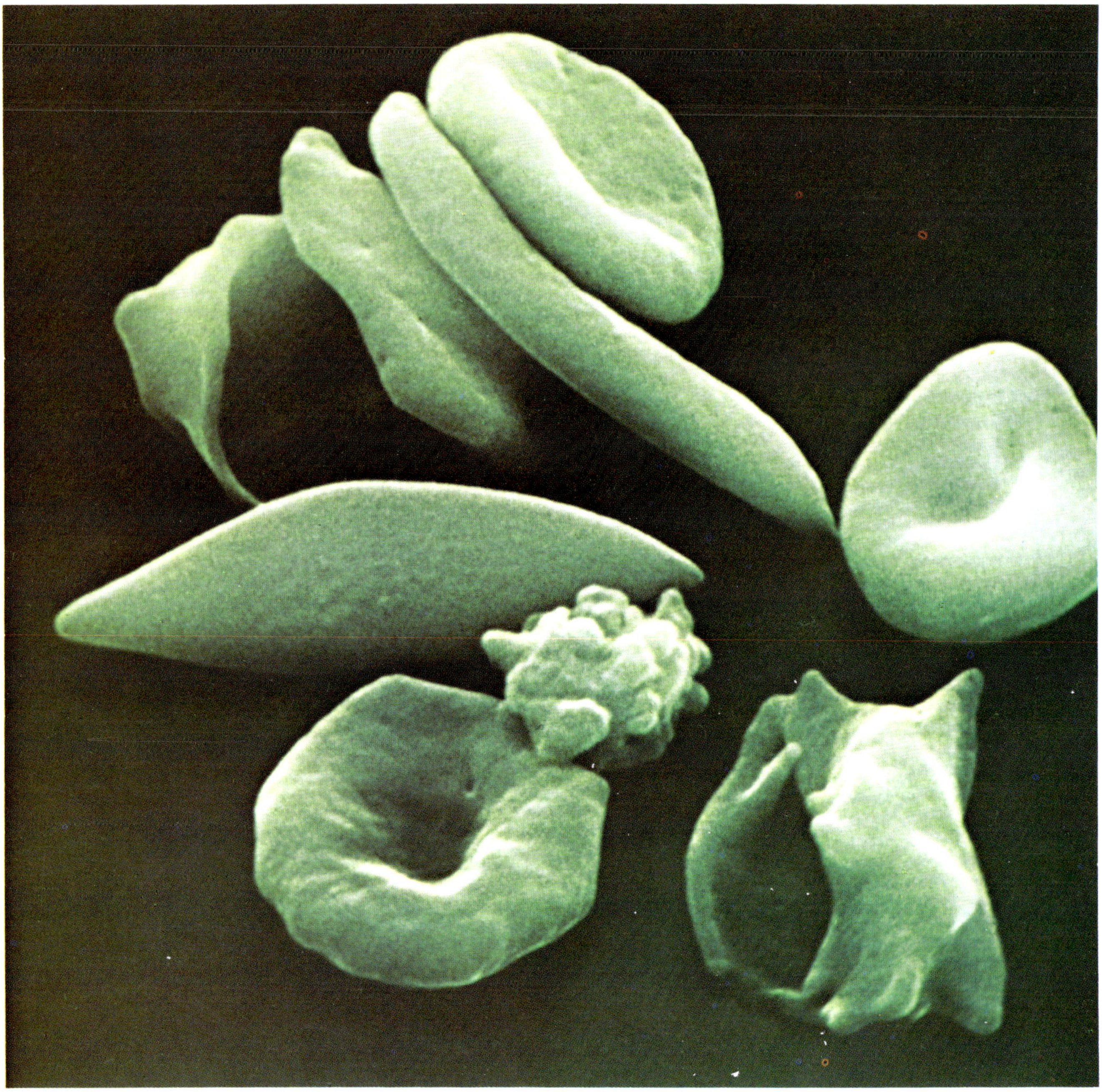

of light microscopy. Generally the pits are shallow, occurring also on Hb S biconcave discs (Fig. 17). Such scars may mark membrane areas occupied by surface projections formed in prior sickling episodes. Pits could signify a resealed area of membrane following projection loss or intracellular retraction on reoxygenation. Also, the pits could be scars left after the RE phagocyte engages in a limited process of surface phagocytosis.

Surface projections may break off or be discarded by the RBC by a process of microbudding or microvesiculation (Fig. 23). The latter process may show itself as single microblebs or as a beaded assembly at the cell surface (Fig. 24). Repeated loss of membrane produces variable sizes of RBC fragments (Fig. 19). Surface area to volume ratio where reduced also results in cell rigidity.

Many of these injured RBC are especially susceptible to permanent entrapment and phagocytosis by reticuloendothelial cells lining splenic and liver sinusoids. Anemia is the outcome whether hemolysis occurs within the circulation from mechanical forces or is intracellular during phagocytosis.

On deoxygenation Hb S, either inside or outside of the cell, polymerizes to form microfilaments. These filaments organize into fibrils or microcables with cell deformation the consequence. Membrane striations may demark internal fibrillar organization. Frequently microcables of Hb S appear adjacent to the RBC membrane and may account for the loss of surface flicker (Fig. 4). When sickling is extreme more of the cell interior is occupied by microcables.

Reoxygenation of sickled cells reverses the microcable formations. The cell interior appears finely granular and relatively homogeneous (Fig. 25). The membrane on the outside shows occasional surface pits. The internal membrane association with Hb S has not been described for the reoxygenated state.

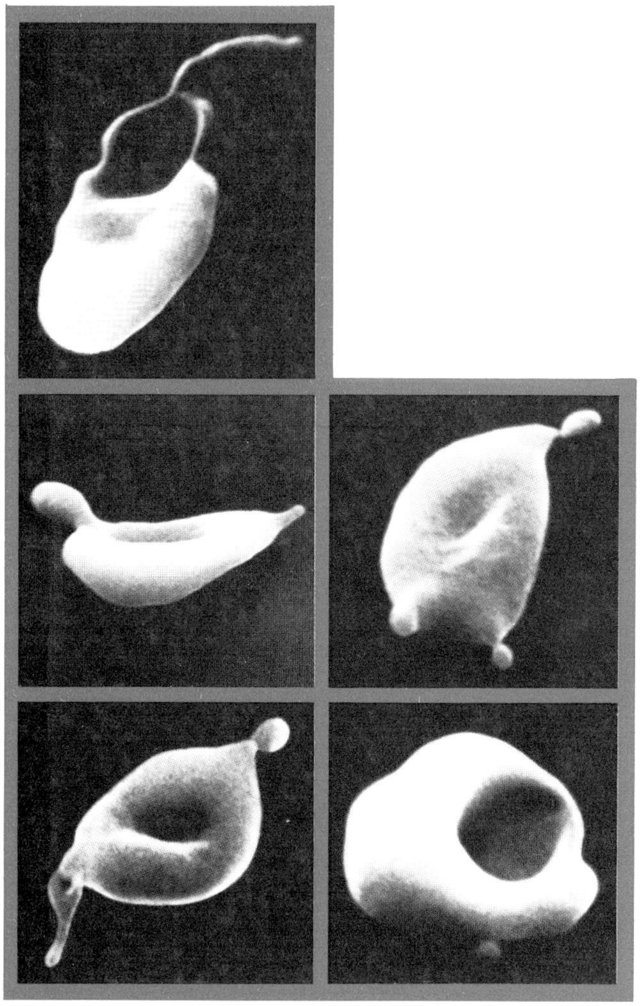

23

24

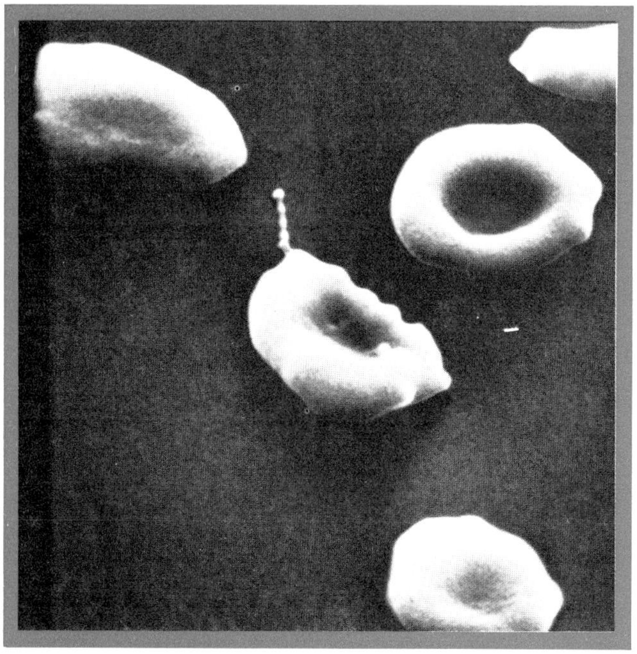

Figure 23. Membrane buds or filaments from RBC of Hb SS subjects viewed by SEM. Such projections can be shed or drawn back into RBC interior (X 8400).
Figure 24. A SEM example of membrane shedding during the desickling of RBC from a Hb SS individual (X 7700).

Figure 25. Comparison of RBC interiors in the sickled and desickled state as viewed by transmission electron microscopy.
A. RBC sickled by chemical deoxygenation with metabisulfite. Note cross-sections of microrods of Hb S in main cell mass and its side projections continuous in other serial sections.
B. Reversal of sickling by addition of urea in invert sugar to above sickled cells. Reversal was about 95% effective in this experiment. Note the interior is fairly homogeneous without Hb S rods visible (X 43000).

A

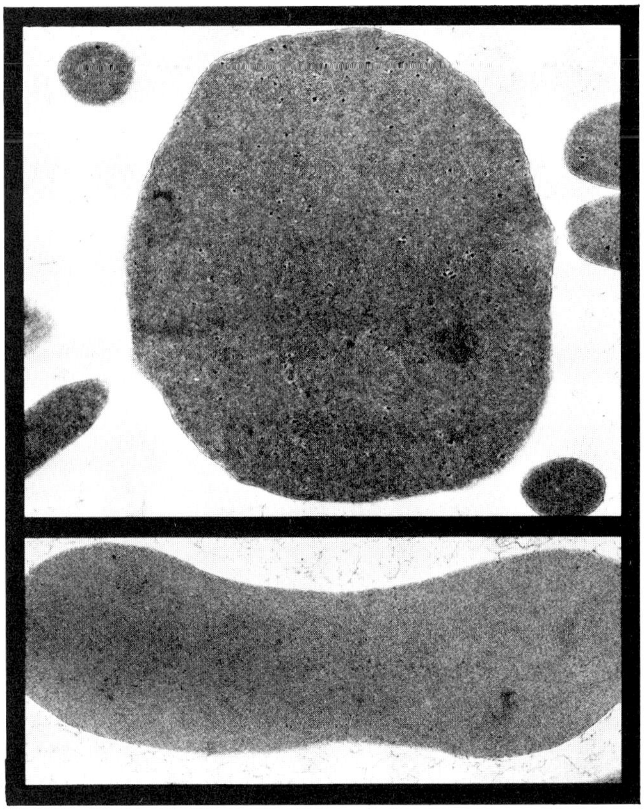

B

ERYTHROCYTE FLEXIBILITY

Some regions of the microcirculation place severe limitations on passage of RBC. To negotiate the narrowest channels (3μ or less in diameter) RBC must deform into various shapes. The biconcave disc shape is the most deformable with more surface area than volume. Sickle cells and spherocytes are poorly deformable and thus become easily trapped.

Erythrocyte rigidity or deformability has been measured in cell suspensions by viscometry, filtration or micropipet. The micropipet technique simulates a capillary which normally is relatively inelastic. Moreover, individual cell visualization and measurements are made and one can determine the relative value of shape versus intrinsic membrane properties for deformability. To negotiate a 14 μ length micropipet of 3 μ diameter, a normal biconcave disc deforms and lengthens about 1.75 fold. With channels of shorter dimension even smaller diameters can be passed as in the spleen.

Flexibility is dependent on the physio-chemical properties of the membrane, on fluidity of the cell contents and on cell shape. While each may vary independently, shape itself is probably the least important determinant.

Intrinsic membrane properties permit almost infinite deformability but restrict stretching to about 15% without cell rupture. ATP has a major role in maintenance of the membrane in its optimum physiologic state. Less than 20% of the ATP energy generated normally by anaerobic glycolysis is used to power the membrane's ion pump necessary for normal salt and water balance. However, only a slight reduction (30%) in normal intracellular ATP concentration stiffens the membrane. As ATP deficiency develops the RBC engages in a disc-sphere transformation. The flexible biconcave disc changes shape to a crenated disc (scallop form), then to a crenated sphere (burr form), and finally to a spherocyte (Fig. 15 and 26). As a governor of membrane flexibility, the chelating property of ATP may be more important than provision of energy. Current thought is that ATP adjusts membrane stiffness by regulating the intramembrane calcium content. Insufficient ATP leaves calcium free to bind to intrinsic membrane proteins thereby decreasing the viscoelastic properties and/or increasing the contractile properties of the membrane. Another important competitive binder for ATP is deoxygenated hemoglobin. Even normal RBC at O_2 tensions below 30 mm Hg exhibit increased rigidity. It is known that excessive intramembrane calcium with concomitant membrane stiff-

Figure 26. Some routes to abnormal erythrocyte deformability and ultimate hemolysis. **A.** ATP deficiency as in the hereditary disorder pyruvate kinase deficiency. Crenated discs (scallops) progress to crenated spheres (burr cells) and ultimately smooth surfaced spheres. **B.** Abnormal hemoglobin as in Hb SS. Oxygen deficiency induces different degrees of sickling. **C.** Oxidative damage and Heinz body formation as in glucose 6 phosphate dehydrogenase deficiency. Ultimately only the RBC membrane with its attached Heinz bodies is left. **D.** Mechanical fragmentation of RBC on obstructions in the blood vessels. **E.** Complement induced membrane damage. Note spiny sphere and hemoglobin extrusion from an immune damaged RBC. **F.** Lipid and lipoprotein defects as in cirrhosis. The bizarre shaped RBC are termed spur cells. **G.** Abnormal membranes as in hereditary spherocytosis. Note wrinkled or honeycombed surfaces and swelling. Membrane loss results in microspherocytes. **H.** Salt and water leakage as in osmotic damage. Biconcave discs swell to regular size spherocytes which may rupture with loss of Hb. Thus holey cells result or membrane remnants (ghosts) or microspherocytes (SEM X 5000).

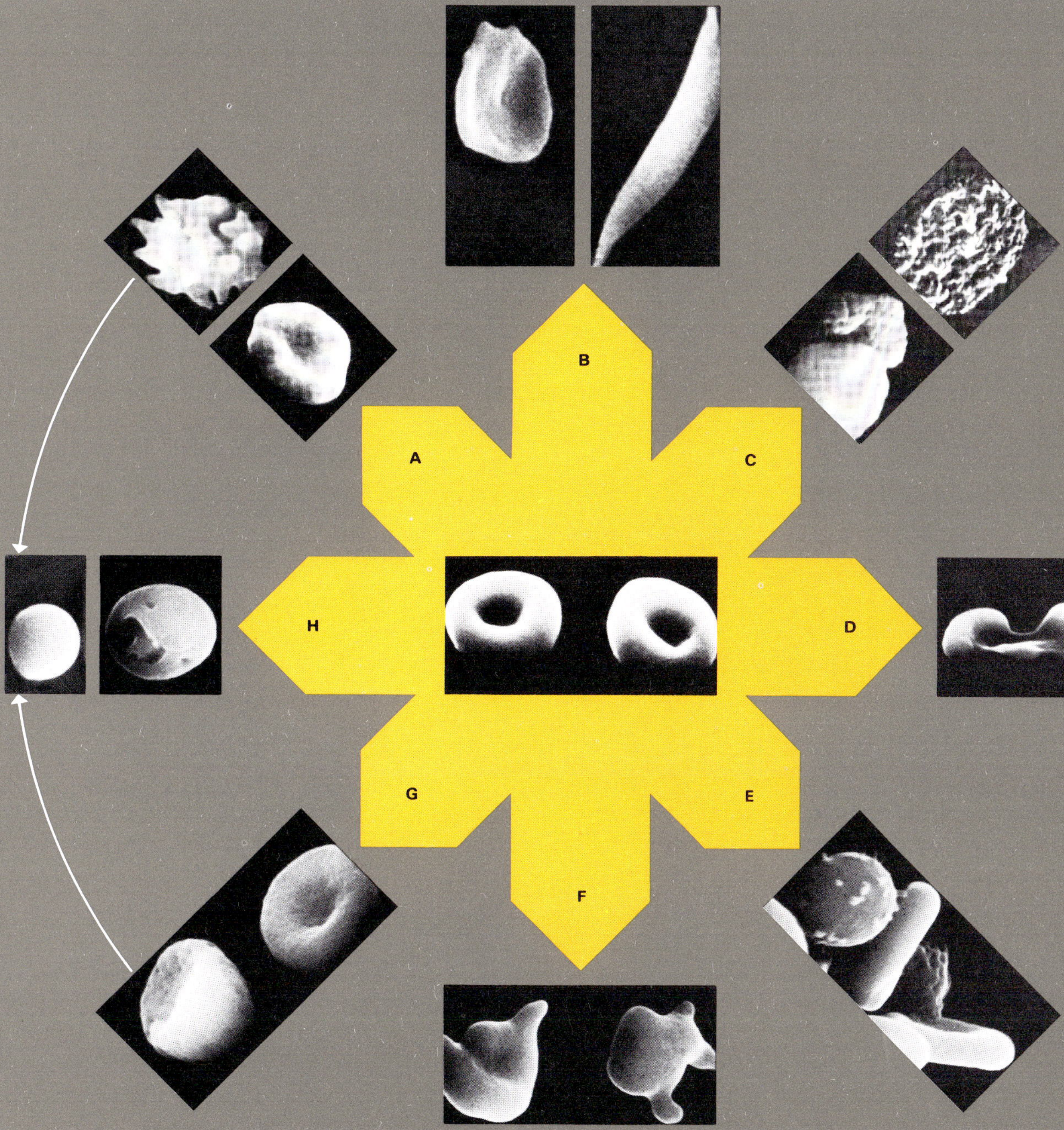

Figure 27. Phagocytosis by macrophages in the splenic cords of the red pulp. SEM of dog spleen. Note intense membrane activity (folds and projections). the top RE cell has a blood cell sticking to its surface. The bottom RE cell has captured a RBC by enclosing it within RE membrane (X 7600).

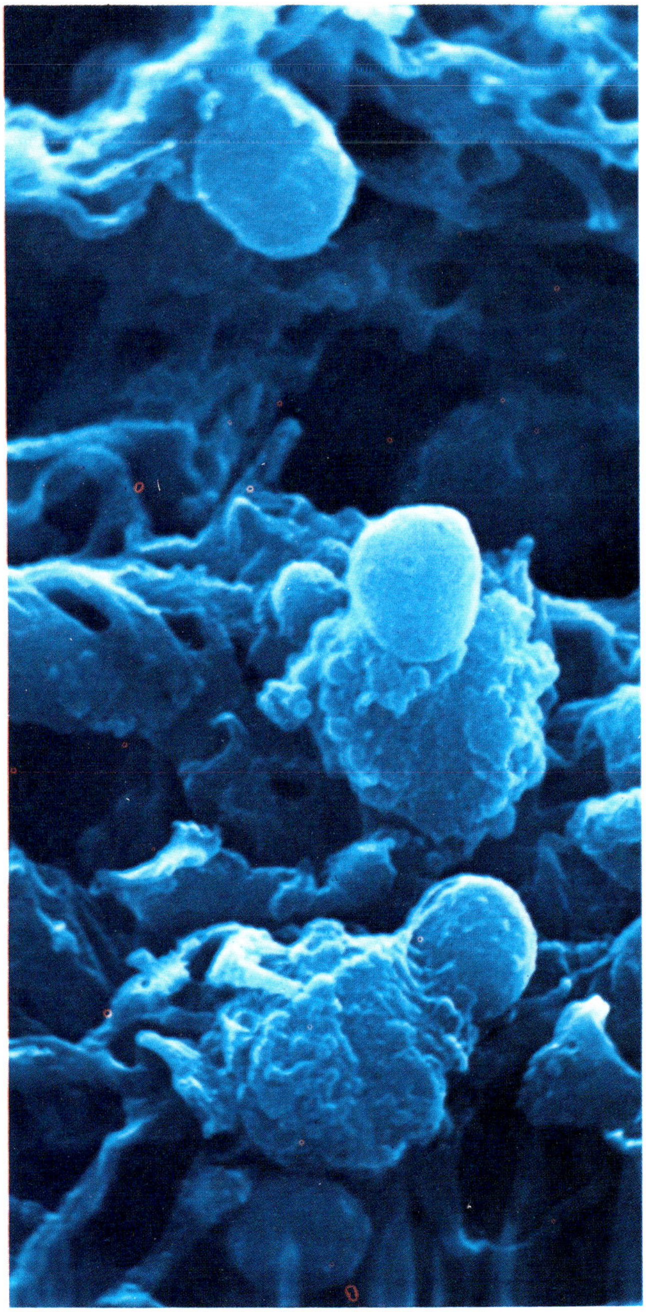

Figure 28. Organization of the red pulp as seen by SEM of dog spleen. The splenic (Billroth) cords surrounding two central blood vessels are seen as reticular meshwork guarded by macrophages. The splenic sinuses appear at the periphery and have openings of various sizes in their wall. Endothelial cell nuclei also are notable within and projecting into the sinus lumen (X 1875).

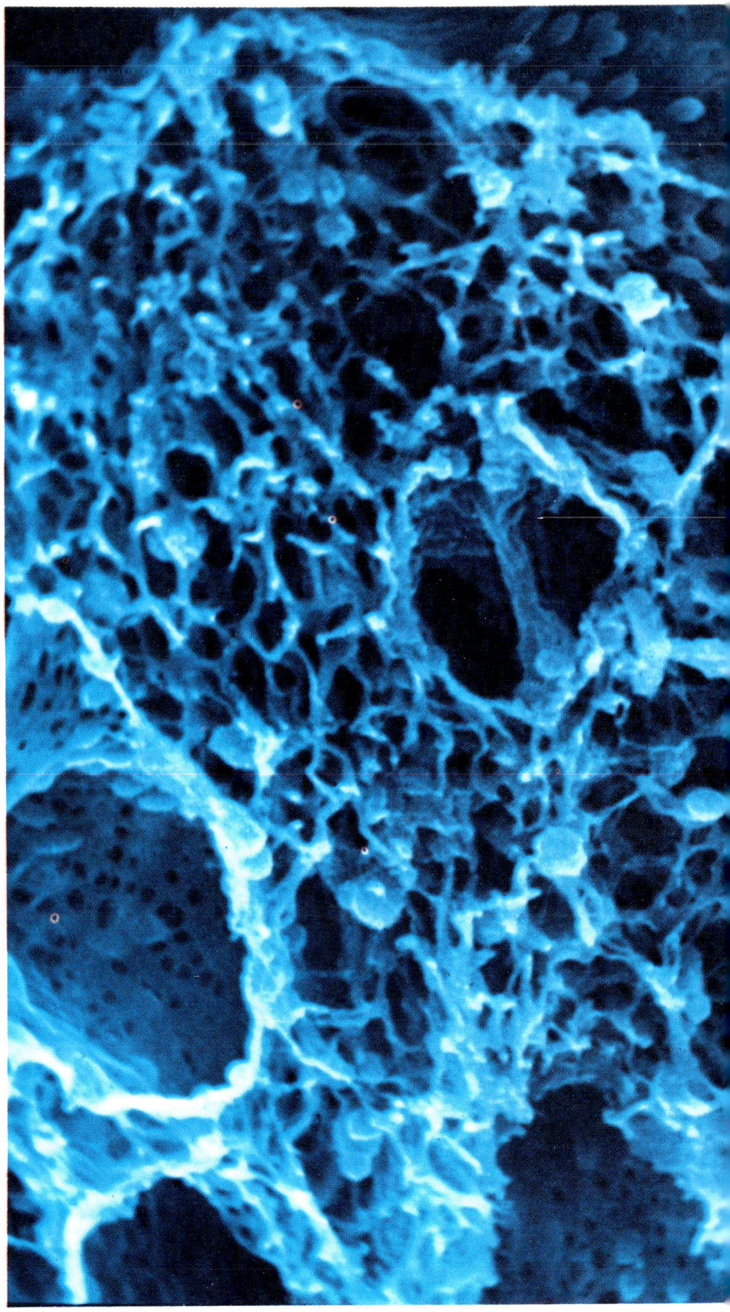

ness can result from either deoxygenated hemoglobin and/or ATP deficiency.

A reduction in fluidity of internal erythrocyte contents also decreases flexibility. The juxtamembrane region is especially prone to hemoglobin aggregation (Fig. 4). In this location shape is readily altered and permanent association with membrane may occur. Examples are stiffened erythrocytes with cargos of Hb S as well as thalassemia cells with denatured hemoglobin existing as Heinz bodies. Hemoglobin C crystal formation also decreases deformability and may even rupture erythrocytes.

ERYTHROCYTE DESTRUCTION

Life span for normal erythrocytes is about 120 days. The anucleate adult cells having shed their nuclei in the bone marrow undergo senescence in the blood. As they age there is denaturation and loss without replenishment of essential enzyme machinery. Membrane maintenance and the proper surface area to volume relation are vital to erythrocyte survival.

Several mechanisms can shorten erythrocyte life, (Fig. 26). In all of these the membrane is of paramount importance. Sphering and/or bizarre forms of increased rigidity occur. Membranes become sticky or lose their ability to repel other cells. There may be actual loss of membrane. Hemoglobin must not necessarily spill into the plasma for a hemolytic state to exist. Some hemoglobin may separate from the cell and remain membrane enclosed. Fragmentation forms (schistocytes) can result. Erythrocyte survival is conditioned by the environment, the degree of membrane injury, or senescence. The terminal stage for most deteriorating red cells is capture and phagocytosis by reticuloendothelial cells (Fig. 27).

Erythrophagocytosis is predominantly located in the spleen and liver. The primary graveyard for injured red cells is in the red pulp of the spleen. The liver usually serves as a secondary graveyard. (An exception is that immune damaged and agglutinated red cells are predominantly sequestered and phagocytized in the liver.)

The spleen has a unique organization of anatomy and circulation. This makes it especially suitable as a sensitive detector of erythrocyte injury and disposal. The most restrictive portion of the circulation is in the red pulp of the spleen. Erythrocytes that are poorly deformable are entrapped or slowed in their passage through an arena of thrashing professional phagocytes (Fig. 27).

The spleen receives about 200 milliliters of blood/min. Although this represents only 3-5% of the total blood volume, the significance lies in the way the blood is processed. The intricate anatomy of the spleen is better understood because of the extensive work of Weiss using transmission electron microscopy. The 3-dimensional features of the splenic filter are impressive when viewed by scanning electron microscopy (Fig. 28).

Let us follow some routes that RBC can take when delivered to the spleen by the splenic arteries. A small part of splenic arterial blood supplies the white pulp or immunologically competent portion of the spleen. Most of the arterial blood is delivered into the splenic filter (the marginal zone and splenic cords of the red pulp). This continuum is a close meshwork of reticular fibers guarded by the RE phagocytes (splenic macrophages). This area provides the intermediate circulatory compartment which is functionally an open circulation. Blood cells in this peculiar "vascular" compartment gain entry into the venous circuit only by finding and passing through openings in the wall of the splenic sinusoids (Fig. 28). Even there circulation may be slow and cells are subject to entrapment by the ever present phagocytes. This blood moves into veins and exits the spleen.

The Circulation

Sickling as it occurs *in vivo* extracts a pathophysiologic toll from the cardiovascular system. Repeated sickling produces a pattern of vascular injury notable in young adults with sickle cell anemia. Although episodic, sickling can reduce the circulation and even obstruct blood vessels to impair organ and tissue function. Such injuries may appear to have an erratic distribution with transient or permanent effects.

Brief consideration of the pertinent basic science of the cardiovascular system should aid understanding of the distribution of sickling injury.

The cardiovascular system is a closed complex of pipes and pumps. This system functions to circulate the blood and to insure that organs and tissues receive an adequate supply of nutrients and have an outlet for their wastes. Circulation is perpetuated by the force of the heart assisted by arterial contractions. Return blood flow is encouraged by venous contraction and unidirectional valves supplemented by the extravascular contraction forces of adjacent muscles.

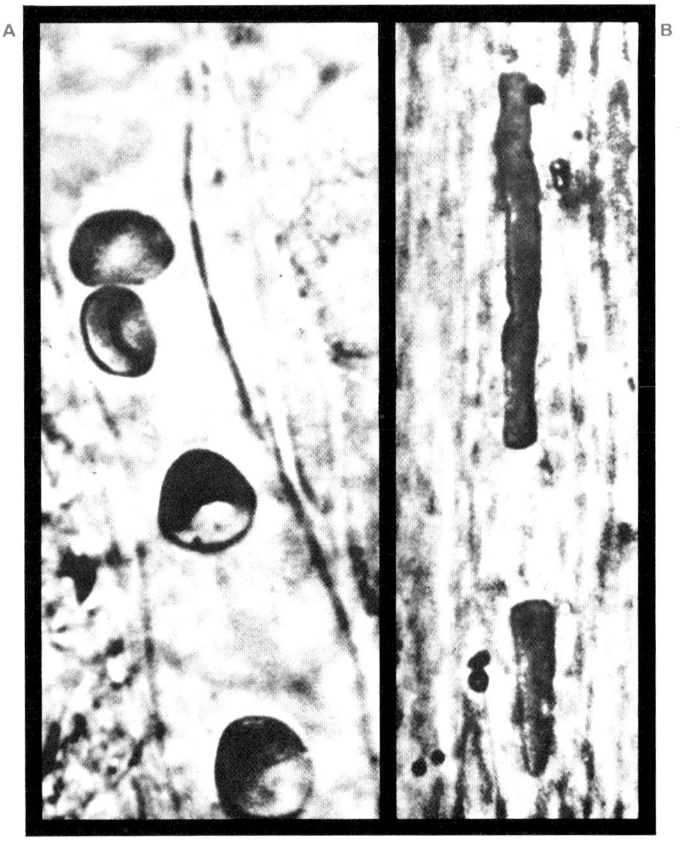

Figure 29. Microcinephotographs of RBC circulating in human vessels of very small caliber. A. Note typical biconcave disc form. B. When vessel is very small the RBC must be very flexible to negotiate the space in single file (X 2500).

The exchange of materials essential for cell activity occurs in the microvasculature. For the adult human with 1.2×10^9 vessels at least 99% comprise the microvasculature (arterioles, capillaries, sinuses, venules). Most capillaries are relatively inelastic and small bore tubes with diameters of 3-16 μ. As a consequence, RBC (diameter near 8 μ) must flow through single file or deform to negotiate the passage. The flexibility or rigidity of RBC becomes of prime importance for blood flow in narrow vessels. Branemark documents spectacularly the extreme deformability of blood cells by ultra high speed cinemicrography of the human microcirculation (Fig. 29).

Capillaries provide enormous areas for transvascular exchange. Although the capillary density and structure varies among the tissues, it is rare for a cell to be farther than 0.1 mm away. Skeletal muscle with its metabolically greater needs has about 2000 capillaries in 1 mm^2 area. At rest about 33% of the total available O_2 is extracted by muscle. But active skeletal muscle extracts about 75% of the O_2. Normally the quantity of microcirculation parallels the organ needs. Brain, heart and skeletal muscle have dense capillary networks to support their active metabolisms. Skin and kidneys also have large blood flows but relatively small amounts of O_2 are extracted for metabolic purposes. The skin flow is largely for heat dissipation. Blood flow through the kidney is largely to purify the blood and form urine.

Within a given capillary the oxygen content and

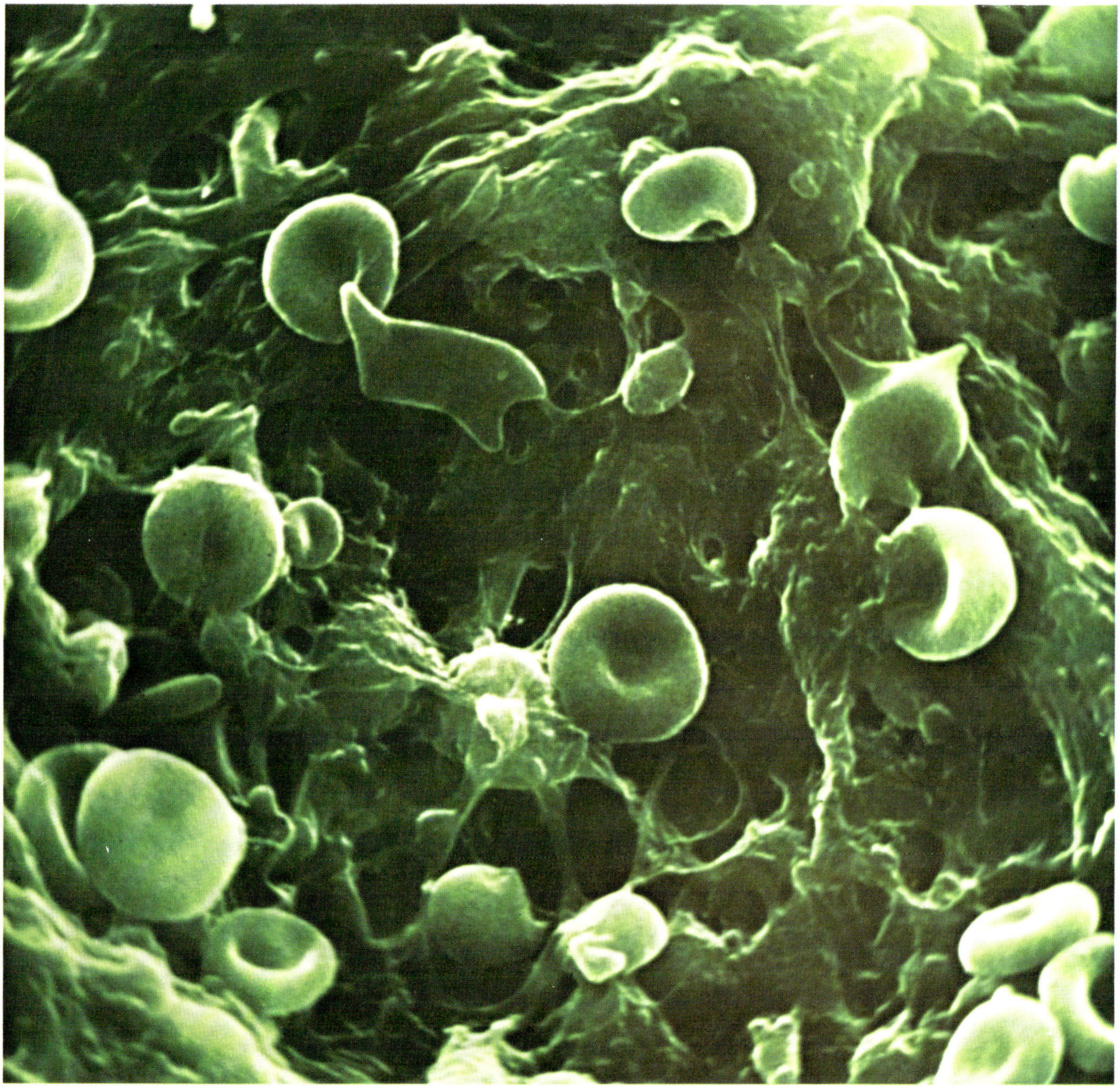

Figure 30. Sickled RBC in red pulp of spleen viewed by SEM. Note size of openings in reticular meshwork. RBC must pass through these and others in splenic sinus to return to the venous circuit (X 6300).

Figure 31. SEM of human spleen to illustrate organization of splenic cords and splenic sinus. One wall of the splenic sinus has been removed to reveal the slit-like and other openings (arrows) between endothelial cells that form the sinus wall. The spindle shaped protrusions are nuclei (En) of endothelial cells (X 8300).

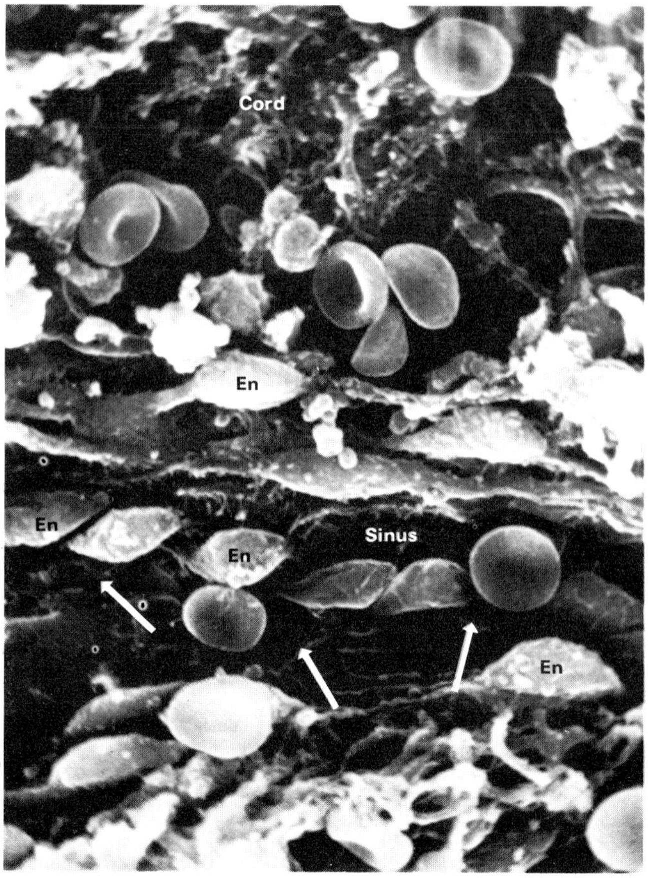

tension decreases as blood flows toward the venule. The magnitude of the depletion relates to how much O_2 is extracted enroute by metabolizing cells. Although arteriolar blood may have a PO_2 of about 100 mm Hg, during capillary transit of a metabolically active organ the PO_2 may drop to 12-17 mm Hg near the venule. Such areas of deoxygenation, if flow is slow, may be lethal corners for Hb SS erythrocytes.

When sickled RBC obstruct within the microcirculation at either the entering arteriole, capillary bed or draining venule, the life lines to adjacent cells are impaired. Minimal cell injury is likely if small regions of the capillary bed are blocked. With venule blockage the back pressure may be sufficient to discourage flow into that capillary bed. Obstruction in arterioles stops circulation into the capillary bed. Fortunately, adjacent channels are often available for blood flow and the demands of the organ can be met.

When damage to the microvasculature is slight or brief the affected individual may not even become aware of vaso-occlusion. The sickling episode may progress, give only transient difficulty, and yet resolve itself without clinical intervention. Sometimes sickling provokes symptoms that are very painful and hospitalization is required. Collateral circulation can develop but requires time.

A vicious sickling cycle may begin with reduced or slow blood flow. The resulting local oxygen deprivation is accompanied by accumulation of acid waste products (i.e. CO_2, lactic acid) which shift the blood pH toward acidity. Exercise and/or infection amplify the tissue asphyxia to provide more sickling signals.

Pain is a response to the tissue injury. It is of variable intensity depending on the extent of involvement and on the ischemic region's location. The ability to bear pain is entirely individual. Frequently, the response to severe pain is to increase muscle activity and mental anxiety. Such responses raise higher the requirements for O_2 while also contributing to the ischemia. Sedation and bed rest reduce the oxygen needs of the patient.

Persistence and extension of the injury can provoke inflammation and lead to permanent organ damage. Moreover, obstruction of blood flow to vital areas of brain, heart or lung may be life threatening.

THE SPLEEN

Blood rheology is particularly significant in the spleen. In this low pressure and low shear rate system of small vessels, cords and sinuses, blood viscosity is increased as hematocrit is increased. Hemoconcentration results from plasma skimming and entrapment of the more rigid RBC that arrive or are produced within the spleen. These factors contribute to the slower circulation and relative stasis in certain areas of the spleen. The abnormal RBC of hemolytic disease exert profound influences here.

Blood flow in the spleen can take a relatively rapid transit or a slow transit route. Normally flexible erythrocytes negotiate the splenic maze with speed similar to their movement through other organs. This is because much of the arterial influx into the red pulp is opposite or near an exit route into the sieve-like area of venous sinuses. Poorly deformable RBC either plug the exit sites or are deflected to wander in the cordal maze (Fig. 30). Thus, senescent and/or injured RBC are liable to all hazards of the splenic environment. The perils encountered may be described as mechanical, metabolic or phagocytic.

The mechanical perils occur at several levels. Small arteries of the spleen have narrow channels as the endothelial cells are high. Mechanically fragile RBC such as sickle cells are squeezed and battered in these passageways. The reticular maze of the marginal zone and splenic cords offer countless sites for mechanical trauma (Fig. 31). Finally the entry openings (some as small as 0.3-0.5μ) into the splenic sinus provide additional opportunities for much cell fragmentation.

The metabolic perils are enhanced by the low pressure and slow circulation especially along the tortuous cordal route. The red pulp is more acidic (pH 6.4 to 6.8) than normal (pH 7.4). The oxygen tension is considerably lower than in most organs and glucose concentration is relatively low. Even normal RBC that linger too long in this area stiffen when PO_2 falls below 30 mm Hg.

Figure 32. Erythrophagocytosis in human spleen as seen by SEM. This RE cell lies free in the splenic sinus. Note the intense membrane activity and that a micro biconcave disc is trapped in a surface pocket of the macrophage (X 9500).

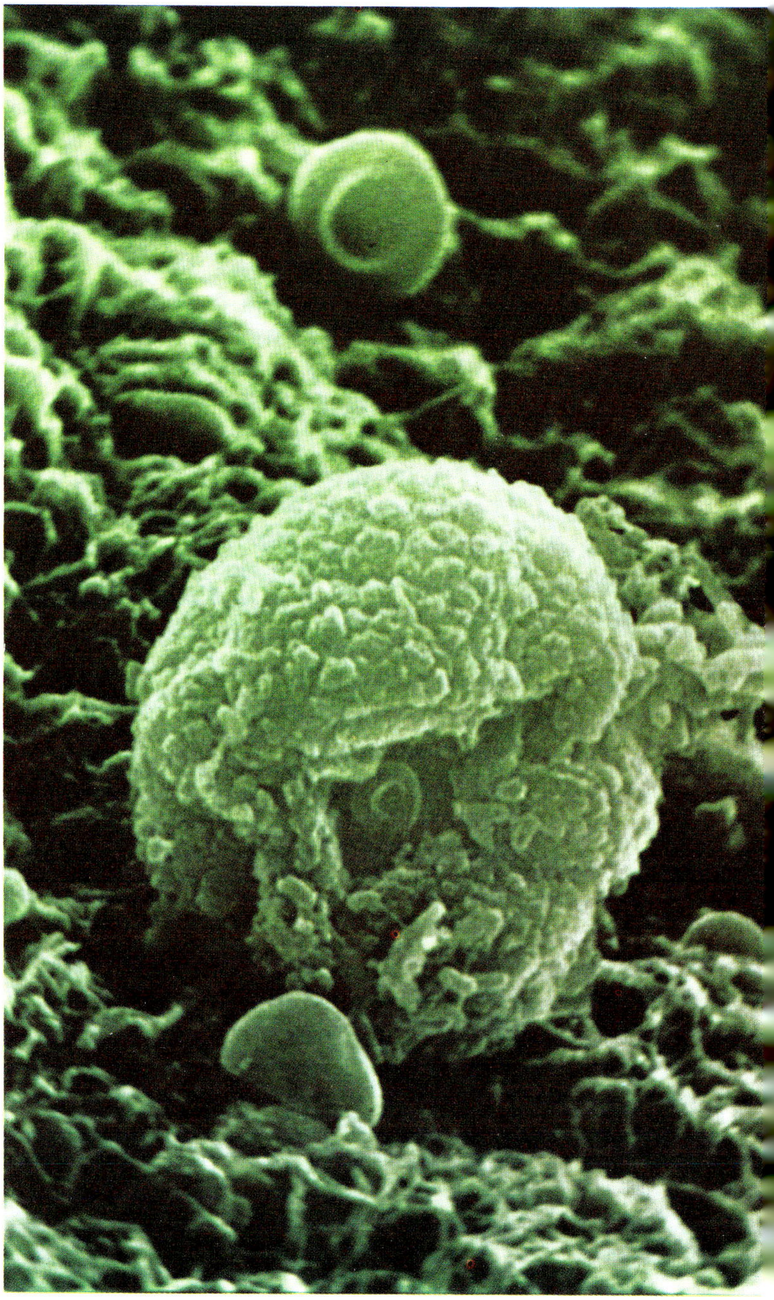

Figure 33. Capture of sickle cells by a Kupffer (phagocytic) cell guarding a sinus (oval shaped) discharging blood into central vein of liver (X-5000).

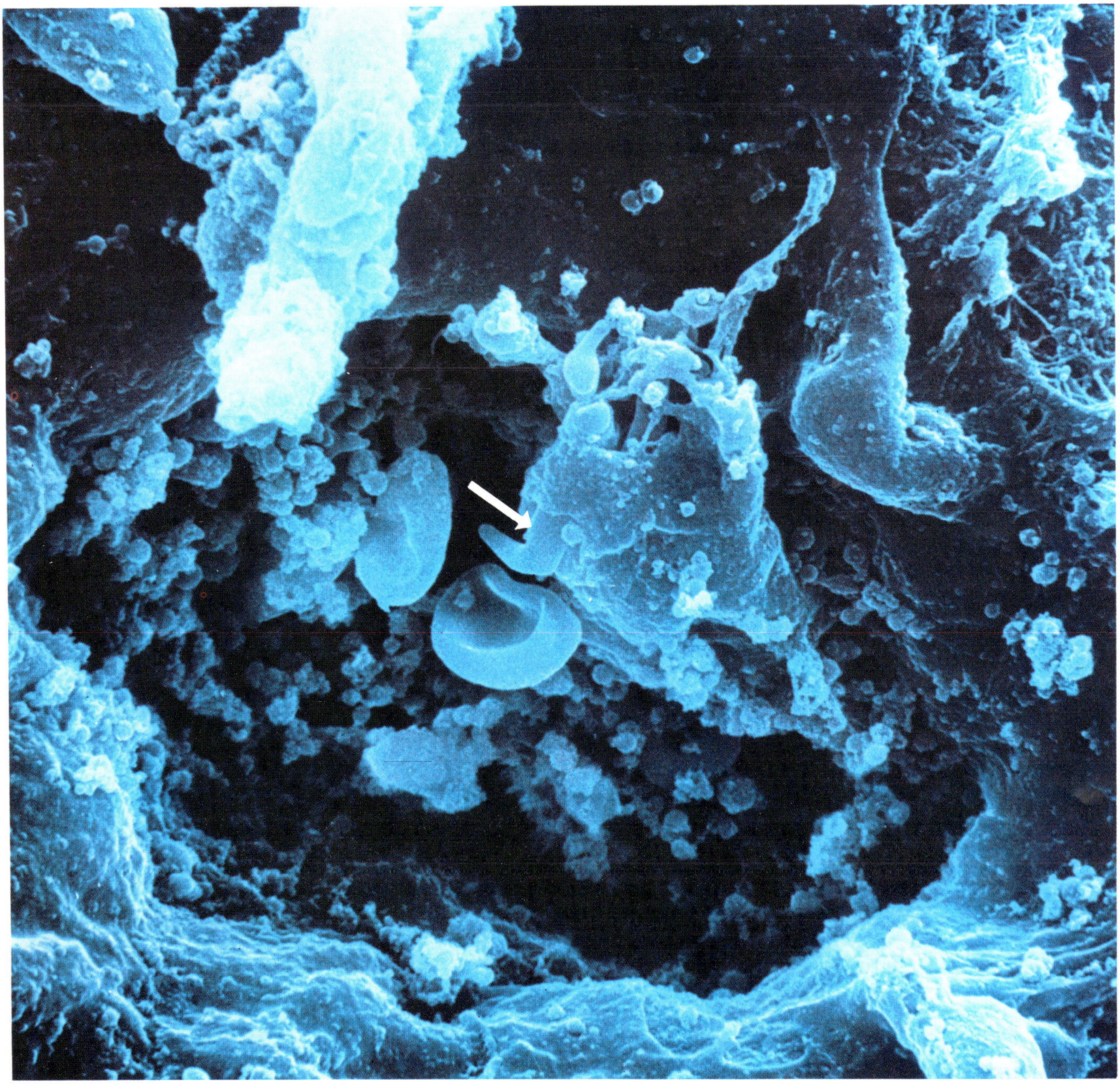

Phagocytic perils are prominent in the cordal area and also within sinuses (Fig. 32). Red cells that are stuck in exit openings or temporarily impaled in the reticular maze are easy prey for the splenic phagocytes (Fig. 27). Partial phagocytosis may occur before RBC are buffeted loose. Complete phagocytosis and intracellular digestion may also occur.

Phagocytic activity in the spleen, of course, may be beneficial. Pitting function is an example and involves partial phagocytosis of localized areas of damaged membrane. Remnants of sickled hemoglobin, crystals of Hb C and denatured globin (Heinz bodies) of thalassemia RBC when adjacent to the surface can be pitted out. Membrane resealing occurs with little loss of cell contents. Small amounts of membrane can be removed in this way with the repaired fully functional cell returning to the general circulation. When too much membrane is removed, cells become spherical and ultimately their loss of plasticity leads to their complete destruction.

Splenic sickling is, in fact, promoted by the natural environment of the spleen. Working together as sickling stimuli are such stressors as stasis, high hematocrit, increased viscosity, increased Hb S concentration in fragmentation remnants, low pH and low PO_2. In most Hb SS individuals the repetitive intrasplenic sickling and local infarction ultimately produce a functional "auto" splenectomy.

The spleen is not essential for life. Moreover, physicians managing certain types of hemolytic disorders (i.e. hereditary spherocytosis or thalassemia major complicated by hypersplenism) may elect removal of the spleen. In such situations, splenectomy reduces erythrophagocytosis and RBC pooling to prolong RBC life span.

The spleen has other functions than RBC destruction that, when lost or reduced, may prove troublesome for people with Hb SS. Platelet numbers are increased in circulating blood because the usual splenic conditioning reservoir for young platelets may not be accessible. Young platelets are more sensitive to thrombogenic stimuli. Also, reduction of the immunologic role of the spleen, residing in the white pulp and macrophage-lymphocytes interaction, may be a significant factor in the increased susceptibility to overwhelming bacterial infections. This problem is especially pertinent in infants and children under 2-3 years as they may not have developed immunity to common bacterial pathogens.

THE LIVER

The liver plays several roles in RBC destruction. Erythrophagocytosis of severely damaged RBC and/or aggregates occurs at this site (Fig. 33). Since the liver is perfused by about 25% of the cardiac output (1250 ml per minute) a considerable amount of blood can be monitored. However, the RE cells lining liver sinusoids are poor sensors of mildly injured RBC and remain disinterested even after splenectomy.

Hepatic functions also include removal of plasma hemoglobin that may result from intravascular hemolysis. In this case it is the liver parenchymal cell that takes up the circulating hemoglobin either bound to haptoglobin or free.

Another very important activity of the liver is the uptake of bilirubin by liver parenchymal cells. Bilirubin is a catabolic product of hemoglobin processing during erythrophagocytosis. The phagocytes release bilirubin into plasma. Jaundice results when plasma bilirubin is not removed in sufficient quantities by the liver (Fig. 39). The liver parenchymal cells excrete a bilirubin glucuronide complex into bile. In hemolytic disorders the liver excretes bile rich in bilirubin. Not uncommonly, bilirubin gallstones occur and their existence and the subsequent inflammation further compromise liver function.

Clinical Picture of Sickle Cell Anemia

According to Murayama's hypothesis, hemoglobin S molecules, when deoxygenated, polymerize by means of hydrophobic interaction to form microfilaments and microcables which result in distortion of the RBC. The resulting sickle forms may then occlude the microcirculation with subsequent infarction and necrosis. Almost all of the clinical manifestations, symptomatology and ultimate progressive disability seen in individuals with sickle cell anemia are the direct result of such vaso-occlusive phenomena.

SYMPTOM SYNOPSIS

The disease is characterized by a chronic hemolytic anemia and intermittent "crises" of variable frequency and severity. The latter include pain crises, other acute vaso-occlusive episodes such as pulmonary or central nervous system infarction, as well as aplastic crises. In addition there is an increased incidence of bacterial infection. A multiplicity of symptoms may occur with gradual involvement of many tissues and organ systems. Life expectancy is reduced —many succumb in infancy or early childhood and most do not survive the 4th decade. The clinical picture is quite variable however, with some remaining relatively asymptomatic for many years while others become severely disabled or die at an early age.

While some features of the disease may be seen at any age (e.g. anemia, painful crises, bone infarcts), others characteristically occur in certain age groups. For example, dactylitis, overwhelming pneumococcal sepsis and acute splenic sequestration crises are most often seen in infants and young children, while leg ulcers, aseptic necrosis of the femoral head and retinal lesions are usually seen in adolescents and young adults.

The infant genetically destined to have sickle cell anemia has no symptoms in the first few months of life due to the protective effect of fetal hemoglobin (Hb F). At birth 50-95% of hemoglobin is Hb F. While individual RBC vary in the amount of Hb F they contain, the majority contain enough Hb F to prevent sickling. After birth the percentage of Hb F drops off at the rate of 3-4% each week. Thus by 4-5 months of age the infants RBC contain predominantly Hb S and are capable of being sickled. From that time on there is a gradual accumulation of problems, the infant being susceptible to all of the sequelae of intravascular sickling.

Clinical manifestations are generally first noted between 6 months and 2 years of age, the most common presenting problems in this age group being infection, dactylitis, severe anemia, colic and irritability. What might be recognized as a pain crisis in an older child may appear as irritability or colic in an infant. Sickle cell dactylitis ("hand-foot syndrome") may be the initial manifestation (Fig. 34). Others may present with a bacterial infection, as pneumonia, with pallor and jaundice being incidental findings on examination. After 6 months of age anemia is a constant finding with hemoglobin values generally ranging between 6-9 gms %. Hepatosplenomegaly is noted in 50-75% of those seen in the first two years, while pallor, scleral icterus and hemic murmurs are noted in approximately 35%.

VASO-OCCLUSIVE CRISES

The clinical course of the disease is characterized by relatively asymptomatic periods alternating with crises. By far the most common type of crises are "pain crises," resulting from local intravascular sickling, stasis and vaso-occlusion. Pain crises in childhood often appear to be preceded by infection, dehydration, acidosis, cold exposure, or unusual stress such as trauma, strenuous physical exertion or emotional disturbance; however in many cases there is no apparent precipitating event. Pain crises vary considerably in frequency, intensity and duration. Although crises may be mild and of short duration often pain is excruciating, necessitating hospitalization and narcotic analgesics. The pain is generally throbbing in nature, may be migratory, and is often accompained by low-grade fever. Hemoglobin and hematocrit values are either unchanged from precrisis values, or are somewhat higher due to dehydration and hemoconcentration (see section on Renal Lesion, p. 51, 52, 53, and 54).

Dactylitis. Dactylitis is often the first manifestation of sickle cell anemia. Resulting from ischemic necrosis of the small tubular bones of the hands and/or feet, it is characterized by soft tissue swelling, heat and tenderness over the metacarpals and proximal phalanges (Figs. 35 and 36). The "hand-foot syndrome" is often bilateral. Although the peak age incidence is 2 years, it may be seen from 6 months to 8 years. Healing occurs spontaneously. Roentgenograms taken at the onset of symptoms reveal soft tissue swelling only, as symptoms precede radiographic bone changes by 7-14 days. In most cases several tubular bones are affected at one time, with infarction and necrosis being followed by subperiosteal new bone formation, expansion of the shafts with cortical thinning, and widening of the intertrabecular spaces with thinning of individual trabeculae (Figs. 37 and 38). Absorption of infarcted areas results in radiolucent zones on x-ray. The contour and structure of the infarcted bones are usually restored completely within several months; however, recurrences are common.

Joint pain, swelling and limitation of motion occurs frequently in children with sickle cell anemia. Usually resulting from juxta-articular infarcts (terminal vessels and poor collateral circulation), such joint symptoms may mimic acute rheumatic fever.

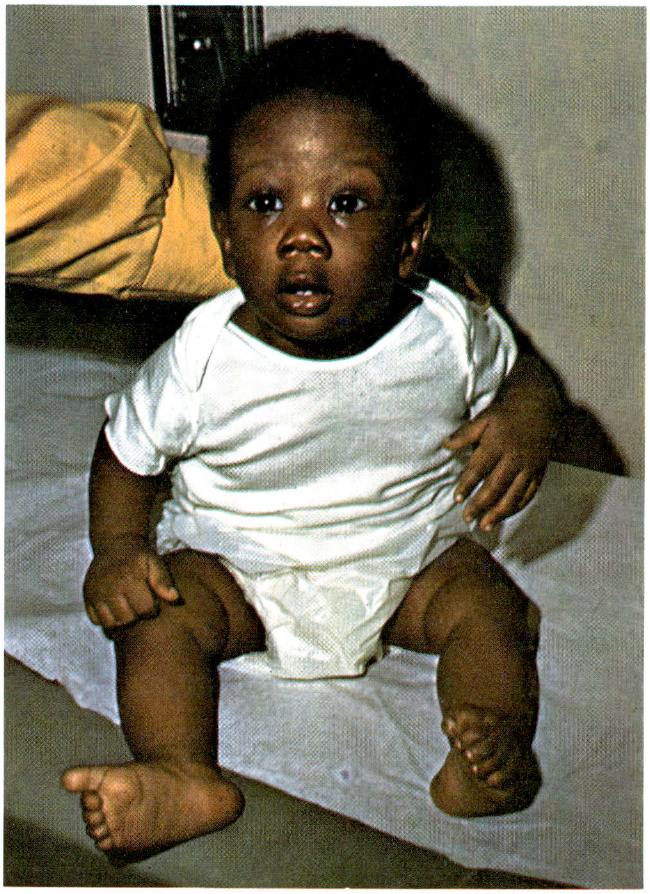
34

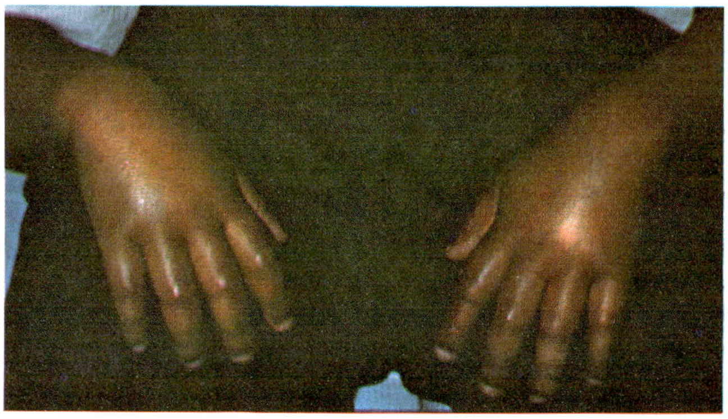
35

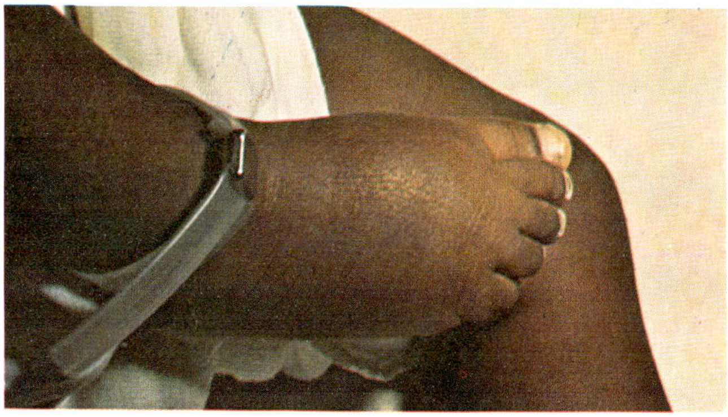
36

Figure 34. Six month old boy who presented with dactylitis as initial manifestation of sickle cell anemia.
Figure 35. Another example of sickle cell dactylitis ("hand-foot syndrome").
Figure 36. Dactylitis involving foot of still another child.

Figure 37. Characteristic roentgenographic features of sickle cell dactylitis. Note **A.** widening of 5th metacarpal bone with periosteal reaction and **B**. similar changes involving 1st and 2nd metacarpals.

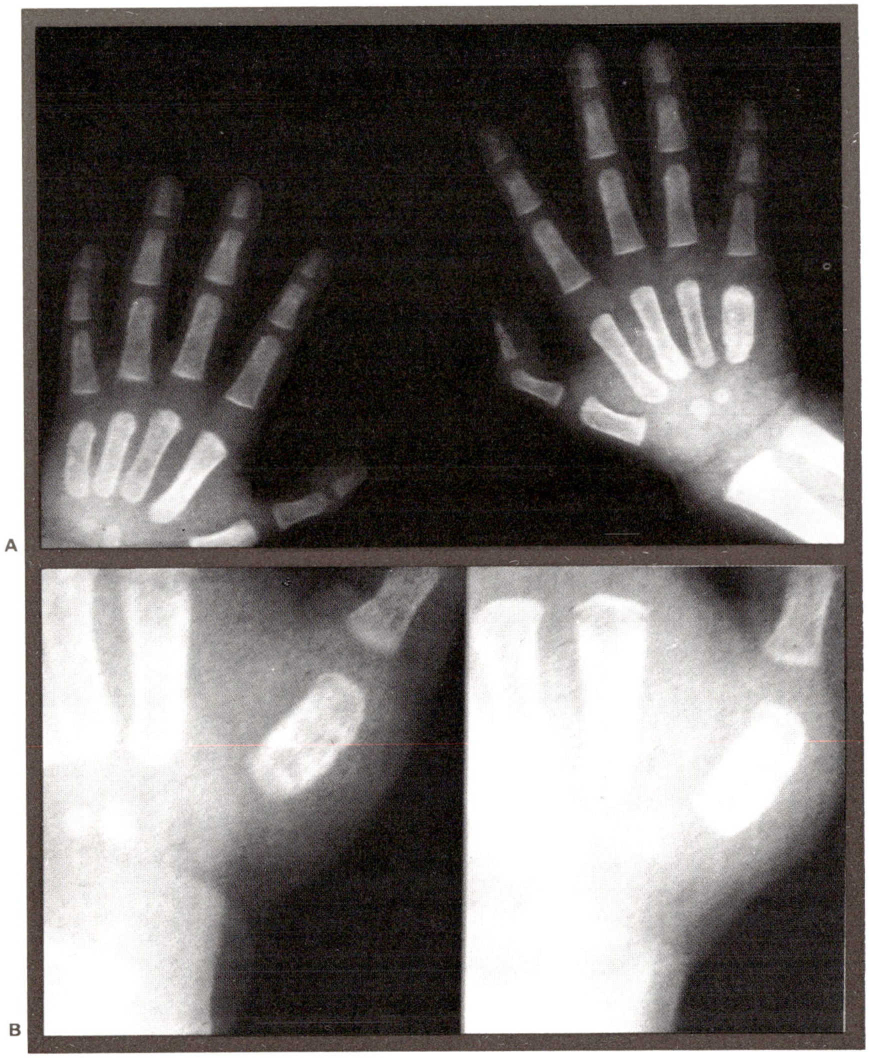

Figure 38. Dactylitis and lead lines in 18 month old child with sickle cell anemia and chronic lead poisoning.

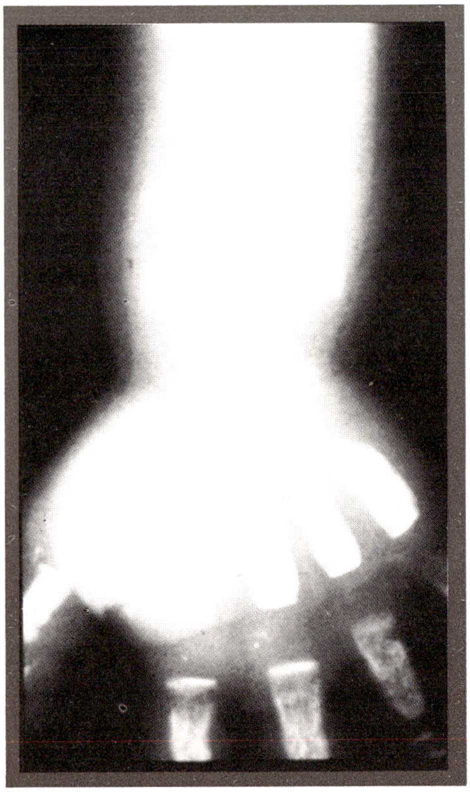

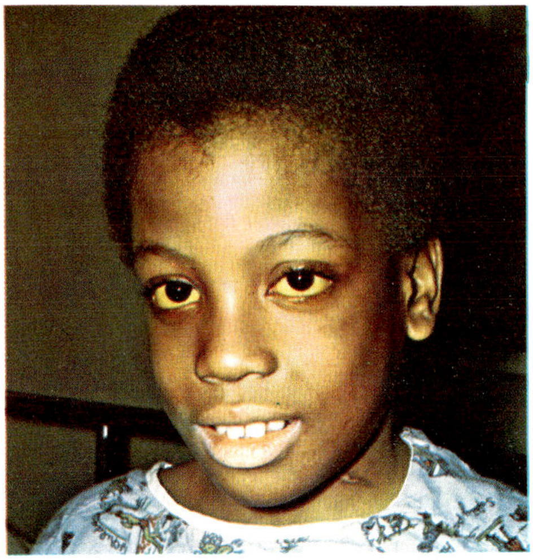

Figure 39. Eight year old boy with sickle cell anemia. Note scleral icterus and prominent forehead.

There is frequently temperature elevation and leukocytosis. Multiple joints may be involved and the pain may be migratory. Joint effusions are seen infrequently in sickle cell anemia. These usually involve the knee or elbow and must be differentiated from septic arthritis.

In children, abdominal pain crises are frequent. The pain is usually diffuse and is often accompanied by fever, tenderness to palpation, and leukocytosis. The clinical picture may simulate acute appendicitis or other surgical abdomen. Abdominal pain crises, as those elsewhere, result from sickling, stasis and vaso-occlusion. In addition to stasis of blood in abdominal viscera, there may be enlargement of the abdominal lymph nodes.

THE SPLEEN

In young children, splenic congestion is common, with some degree of splenomegaly being apparent on roentgenograms as well as by palpation. Splenomegaly usually persists until 5 or 6 years of age but is uncommon thereafter, as repeated infarcts gradually result in fibrosis and scarring. The spleen thus undergoes progressive destruction and diminution, finally becoming a small atrophic siderotic nubbin. The presence of an enlarged spleen after 7 or 8 years of age should make one suspect SC hemoglobinopathy or S-thalassemia rather than sickle cell anemia.

Other distinctive pathophysiologic processes in the spleen are discussed in greater detail in Chapter VI. A state of "functional asplenia", characterized by a bypassing of the reticuloendothelial elements of the spleen, contributes to the increased incidence of overwhelming infections in young children with sickle cell anemia. Acute splenic sequestration (sudden pooling of blood in the spleen) may result in severe anemia, vascular collapse, and even death in some young children.

THE LIVER AND BILIARY TRACT

The liver is usually somewhat enlarged and firm. Tissue sections reveal sinusoidal congestion with sickled RBC as well as varying degrees of degenerative changes and hemosiderin granules in hepatic parenchymal cells. There are several unique features of the microcirculation in the liver as related to sickle cell anemia. Portal vein blood, which supplies about 75% of the blood to the liver, has a lower PO_2 than arterial blood, thus predisposing to sickling. There is an extensive opportunity for RBC to encounter the RE elements (Kupffer cells) lining the liver sinusoids (Fig. 33). Kupffer cells are stuffed with sickled RBC and hemosiderin granules, and there appears to be some degree of obstruction to sinusoidal blood flow by these enlarged Kupffer cells. Slight elevations of unconjugated serum bilirubin are commonly seen in sickle cell anemia and are often manifested by slight scleral icterus (Fig. 39). In addition, approximately 10% of patients have jaundice of the intrahepatic type with elevation of direct-reacting (conjugated) bilirubin and bile in the urine.

Superimposed liver disease may result from serum hepatitis (usually manifested by increased jaundice, hepatic tenderness, nausea and vomiting, as well as elevation of liver enzymes, SGOT, SGPT, and LDH) or focal hepatic necrosis. Sequelae include nodular or diffuse fibrosis.

The chronic hemolysis in sickle cell anemia predisposes to cholelithiasis. Gallstones occur not infrequently in the second decade and are quite common by the third decade. The recognition of acute biliary tract disease may be quite difficult. A clinical picture simulating cholecystitis with right upper quadrant abdominal pain, nausea and vomiting, fever and leukocytosis may occur in abdominal pain crisis in the absence of biliary tract disorder. While serum bilirubin levels of 1-4 gms % are common in sickle cell anemia, the bilirubin is primarily unconjugated (indirect reacting), reflecting increased hemolysis. If conjugated (direct reacting) bilirubin is also increased, some form of biliary obstruction should be considered. Extrahepatic obstruction by calculous disease must be differentiated from intrahepatic disease. A flat plate of the abdomen will reveal radiopaque gallstones (Fig. 40); however, special contrast studies must be employed to demonstrate non-opaque calculi. Gallbladder visualization by oral or I.V. cholecystography is rarely successful if the total serum bilirubin exceeds 5 mgm %. Extrahepatic obstruction may be demonstrated in these patients by percutaneous transhepatic cholangiography, the findings of dilated biliary ducts is usually indicative of common duct obstruction by calculi.

HEMATOLOGIC MANIFESTATIONS

The Anemia. Sickle cell anemia is characterized by a partially compensated hemolytic anemia, hemoglobin values usually stabilizing between 6-9 gms %. While the life span of normal or sickle trait RBC in the circulation is approximately 120 days, the homozygous state is associated with a marked shortening of RBC survival time. Hemolysis results from the intracorpuscular defect; irreversably sickled cells suffer preferential destruction. RBC destruction in all probability results from cumulative mechanical damage following repeated sickling, and from prolonged stasis in such areas of sluggish circulation as the splenic sinusoids.

One method for determining RBC survival time consists of labeling of RBC with radioactive chromium (^{51}Cr) and reinjecting them into the subject's circulation. By this method the half time (T-1/2) of RBC survival in individuals with sickle cell anemia ranges from 3-11 days as compared to 30-33 days in normal subjects. Splenic size, however, appears to influence results, patients with splenomegaly having shorter survival times (T-1/2 3-5 days). These lower values probably reflect splenic sequestration (holding) in addition to actual RBC destruction. Without the splenic component ^{51}Cr T-1/2 ranges from 8-11 days. By localization of the radioactive tag it has been demonstrated that both liver and spleen are active in removal of homozygous S erythrocytes.

Despite the shortened RBC life span, increased RBC production (4-5x normal) enables the patient to maintain a relatively constant hemoglobin of 6-9 gms %. The hyperplastic bone marrow involves almost the entire skeleton, with red marrow remaining in the shafts of long bones throughout life. The increased rate of effective erythropoiesis is reflected by an elevated reticulocyte count (5-25%) and by polychromatophilic RBC on peripheral smear.

In most other types of anemia, compensation for the oxygen flow deficit is corrected by several mechanisms, that is increased cardiac output, redistribution of blood supply and increased erythrocyte 2,3-diphosphoglycerate. In sickle cell anemia the major effective compensatory mechanism is increased cardiac output.

Several possible explanations merit attention as contributing to the lack of compensation by the other two mechanisms in individuals with sickle cell anemia. Redistribution of blood flow is opposed by sickling tendencies in low flow areas of the microvasculature. Shunting of rigid and sickled RBC into larger vessels actually diverts O_2 supply from the tissues. Thus some vascular beds may be perfused predominantly by plasma containing its normal but inadequate supply of dissolved O_2. Tolerance of most types of anemia is influenced by the amount of 2,3 diphosphoglycerate (DPG) within the RBC: i.e. increased DPG facilitates O_2 release from hemoglobin.

Figure 40. Radiopaque gall stones, *fish vertebrae* and widened ribs with coarse trabeculae in 16-year-old girl with sickle cell anemia.

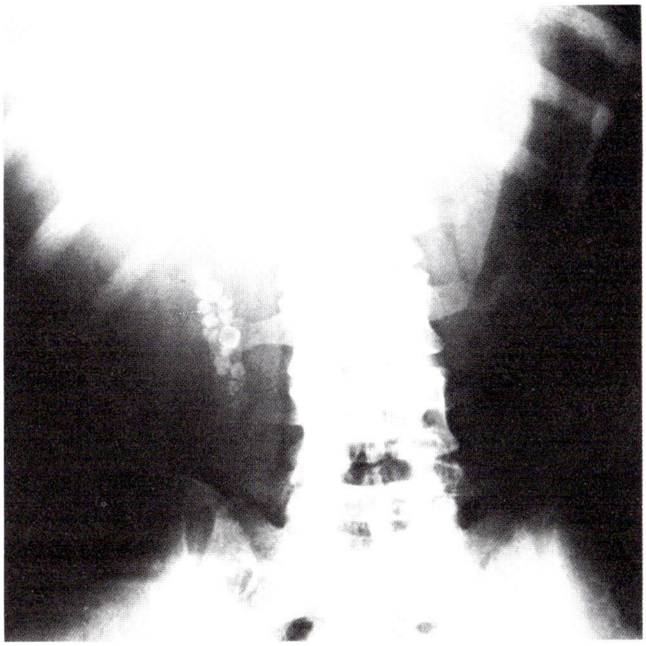

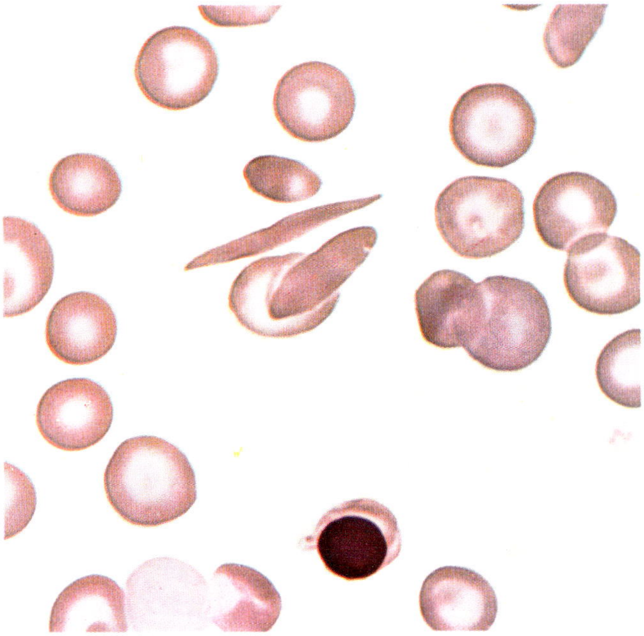

Figure 41. Characteristic peripheral blood smear from child with sickle cell anemia. Note extreme sickled forms as well as target cells, hypochromia and polychromasia.

Paradoxically in Hb SS subjects, even with their increased DPG levels (from reticulocytosis as well as from the fact that Negroes have 15-20% higher DPG levels than Caucasians), there is poor tissue oxygenation. However, there is heterogeneous intracellular distribution and proportionality of DPG, Hb S and Hb F which probably have relevance to the finding of low O_2 affinity of Hb SS whole blood.

The Peripheral Blood Picture. The peripheral blood smear stained with Leishman-Giemsa or Wright's stain characteristically shows a varying number of sickled forms (Fig. 41). There is anisocytosis, poikilocytosis and polychromasia, as well as target cells and occasional nucleated RBC. The bone marrow responds nonspecifically to the increased RBC destruction, with outpouring of increased numbers of WBC and platelets as well as RBC. Thus the leukocyte count generally ranges between 10,000 and 20,000/mm^3, and the platelet count is often elevated as well. These normally elevated WBC values must be kept in mind when evaluating the sick patient.

Other Laboratory Values. The sedimentation rate is slow even in the presence of marked anemia because of the abnormal shape of the sickle cells and poor rouleaux formation. Osmotic fragility is decreased, as the Hb S erythrocytes, poorly filled with hemoglobin, can take up more water before becoming spherical and lysing. Serum haptoglobin values remain very low, as the result of chronic hemolysis, and serum bilirubin (mainly unconjugated) ranges from 1-4 gms %.

Blood Coagulation and Platelets. The standard coagulation screening tests (Quick prothrombin time, partial thromboplastin time and thrombin time) are normal in sickle cell anemia unless complicated by hepatocellular disease. However most patients have elevated platelet counts and factor VIII activity, and during acute pain crises plasma fibrinogen levels are usually increased as well. There is also some impairment of fibrinolytic activity, as manifest by prolonged euglobulin lysis times in the majority of patients studied. In addition, platelet hyperactivity is clearly evident in individuals with sickle cell anemia.[17] While these aberrations may provide a favorable environment for the occurrence of vascular occlusion in the microcirculation, at present one can only speculate on whether or not they play a significant role in the pathogenesis of vaso-occlusive episodes.

Aplastic (Aregenerative) Crises. Although much less frequent than pain crises, *aplastic crises* are the most common hematologic crises seen in sickle cell anemia. Similar aplastic (aregenerative) crises may be seen in individuals with other chronic hemolytic states, as hereditary spherocytosis. These crises are characterized by a rapidly developing anemia due to the cessation of RBC production while excessive RBC destruction continues. Hemoglobin values may drop to 2-3 gms %, and the patient develops increasing pallor and weakness. Aplastic crises often occur in the wake of an infectious illness such as viral gastroenteritis or flu-like syndromes, and if there are several children with sickle cell anemia in the household, all may be affected. During the early phase of an aplastic crisis there is reticulocytopenia and the bone marrow is devoid of RBC precursors beyond the pronormoblast stage (Fig. 42). The process is self-limiting, with effective RBC production manifest by reticulocytosis returning in 7-10 days.

Laboratory findings vary depending on the stage of the aplastic crisis (Fig. 43). Often by the time the patient develops weakness and pallor, the hemoglobin and hematocrit values are very low but reticulocytosis may have resumed. Leukopenia of varying

Figure 42. Bone marrow during an aplastic (aregenerative) crisis, showing a predominance of basophilic erythroblasts.

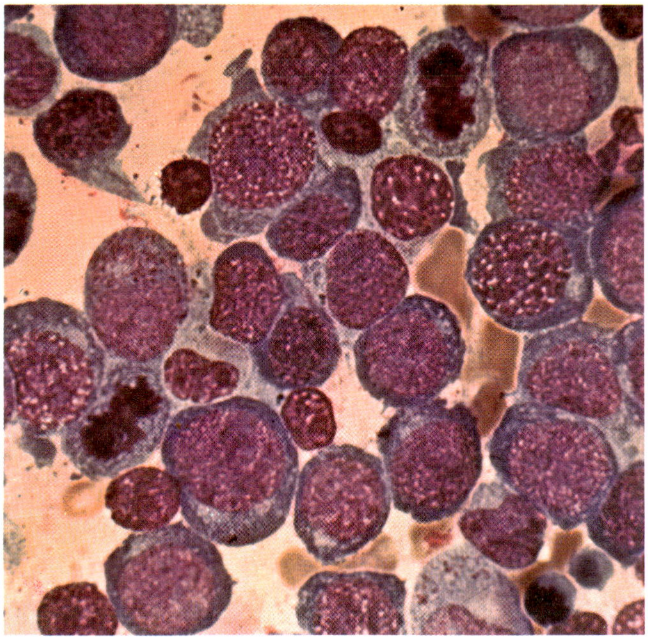

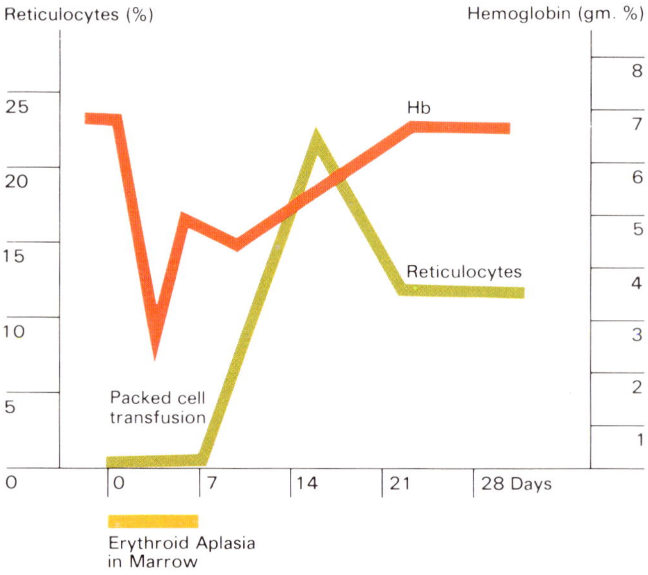

Figure 43. Reticulocyte counts and hemoglobin values during an aplastic (aregenerative) crisis.

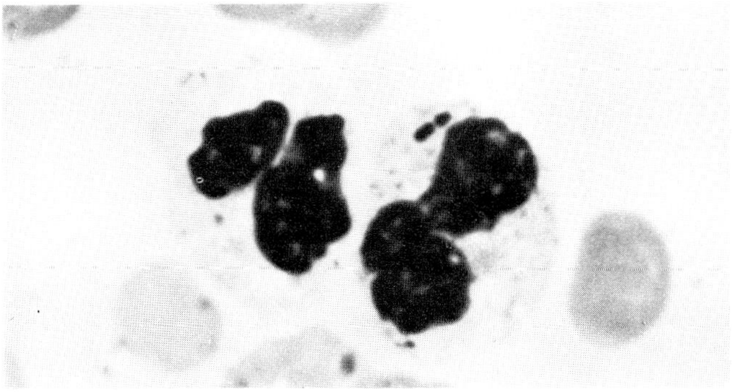

Figure 44. Intracellular diplococci *(D. pneumoniae)* in peripheral blood smear from one year old child with sickle cell anemia.

degrees may accompany an aplastic crisis, but thrombopenia is rarely seen.

Megaloblastic Anemia. Megaloblastic anemia is uncommon in sickle cell anemia, but may occur in pregnancy (where there are excessive demands for folic acid) or in those individuals with very poor dietary intake of folic acid. It is manifest by a falling hemoglobin, increasing pallor and fatigue. Symptoms and signs of congestive heart failure may also be present. Laboratory findings include hemoglobin values of 3-5 gms %., macrocytes, megaloblastic nucleated RBC and hypersegmented neutrophils on peripheral smear, and characteristic megaloblastic changes in the bone marrow. Serum folic acid is low while vitamin B_{12} levels are usually normal.

Hyperhemolytic Crises? The existence of "hyperhemolytic crises," with a drop in hemoglobin resulting from a rapid increase in the rate of RBC hemolysis, has been challenged. While there are a few examples which appear well documented in the literature, such a phenomenon is no doubt rare.

Acute Splenic Sequestration Crises. These episodes are fortunately not common, but are definitely life-threatening! Occurring predominantly in infants and young children, acute splenic sequestration is characterized by sudden severe anemia and hypovolemic shock resulting from sudden massive trapping of RBC within the splenic sinusoids. The clinical features include a rapid increase in pallor and polydipsia, abdominal distention, nausea and vomiting. Dyspnea, weakness and left-sided abdominal pain soon follow, as well as fever and jaundice. Peripheral vascular collapse rapidly ensures, and the child may be dead on arrival in the emergency room only a few hours after the onset of symptoms. In such cases post-mortem findings include generalized vascular engorgement of abdominal viscera, particularly the spleen. In those who arrive at the hospital alive, physical examination generally reveals a shocky patient with marked pallor, jaundice and a rigid abdomen. Convulsions may occur as a result of acute anemic hypoxia, and hemoglobin values of 1-3 gms % are common.

Although some episodes of acute splenic sequestration seem to be precipitated by infection, the etiology remains unknown. It occurs primarily in children between 6 months and 3 years, presumably because their splenic sinusoids are freely distendable (in contrast to older children and adults whose spleens have become fibrotic and scarred). In those who survive there is a tendency for recurrent episodes.

INCREASED SUSCEPTIBILITY TO BACTERIAL INFECTION

Bacterial infection is a major cause of morbidity and mortality in sickle cell anemia, particularly in infants and young children. Sickle cell anemia may be first detected as an incidental finding in young children hospitalized for bacterial infection and such children are unusually susceptible to overwhelming septicemia. Bacterial pneumonia is the most common infection for which patients are hospitalized. In addition some physicians have documented a 300-fold greater incidence of bacterial meningitis (particularly pneumococcal and influenzal) and a 25-fold greater incidence of salmonella osteomyelitis.

The pneumococcus is the most common offending organism in bacteremia (Fig. 44) and meningitis in sickle cell anemia. The majority (80-85%) of these pneumococcal infections occur in children under 3 years of age. While *H. influenzae* is responsible for most cases of bacterial meningitis in all children under 3 years of age, the pneumococcus accounts for 70% of cases in children with sickle cell anemia in this same age group.

Figure 45. Bone changes resulting from Salmonella osteomyelitis in 3 year old child with sickle cell anemia. Note A. radiolucent defect. B. periosteal elevation and areas of sclerosis in the femoral shaft.

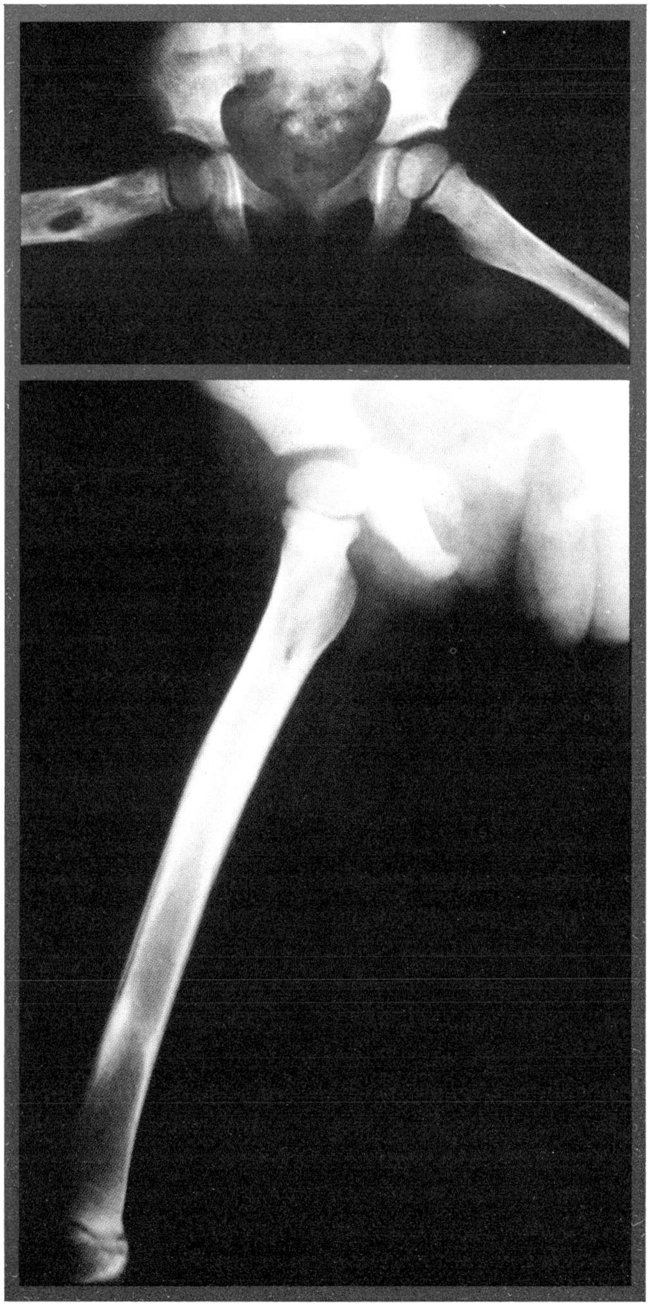

While this unique susceptibility to bacterial infection—particularly pneumococcal infection—has long been recognized, the reasons for it are complex and only partly understood at present. Pneumococci and other pyogenic organisms (as staphylococci, *H. influenzae* and beta hemolytic streptococci) usually invade the body via the respiratory tract. In patients with sickle cell anemia, pulmonary congestion, fluid filled alveoli and areas of infarction no doubt provide an excellent focus for bacterial multiplication and at the same time may impair surface phagocytosis. Many observers have noted the similarity of young children with sickle cell anemia to those children who have been splenectomized early in life, namely their unusual susceptibility to overwhelming bacterial infections. Increased numbers of Howell-Jolly bodies, nuclear remnants normally pitted out in the spleen, was another feature common to both splenectomized and sickle cell anemia subjects. The spleen is quite important in host defense early in life. It not only provides an anatomic site for interaction of immunologically competent tissue with bacterial antigens, but also a slow sinusoidal circulation lined with macrophages capable of clearing bacteria and other foreign particles. It has now been conclusively shown that there is a compromise of splenic phagocytic function in individuals with sickle cell anemia. This so-called "functional asplenia" probably results from sludging of sickled RBC in the microcirculation of the spleen. Sluggish circulation within the splenic cords, low PO_2 and low pH result in sickling, the sickled cells obstruct blood flow through the splenic sinusoids and A-V shunting results. Thus the macrophage-lined sinusoids of the splenic pulp are bypassed. While older children have type-specific antibodies by virtue of previous exposure to pneumococci and are thus able to trap organisms at extrasplenic sites, splenic function appears to be necessary for host response to pneumococci in the absence of preformed antibodies. In the young child with sickle cell anemia the spleen's important role of clearing bacteria from the circulation of the non-immune individual is largely inoperative.

In addition, it appears that serum from persons with sickle cell anemia does not enhance pneumococcal phagocytosis as well as normal serum does. This defective opsonization cannot be attributed to a lack of complement components, as C1, C4, C2 and C3 and present in normal concentrations. Infants and young children are more likely to lack specific antibody to the many antigenic types of pneumococci and other organisms. When specific antibody is deficient, an alternate pathway—the properdin pathway—is used. The properdin system can be activated by bacterial polysaccharides (in the absence of antibody) to fix C3 directly to the bacterial surface, thus promoting phagocytosis. While the sequential interaction of proteins comprising the properdin system is complex and not completely understood, it has been reported that at least some sickle cell anemia patients have a defect in the properdin system which may account for their defective capacity to opsonize bacteria.

Although not nearly as common as pneumonia or meningitis, osteomyelitis is also seen with increased frequency and occurs at all ages (Fig. 45). No doubt bone infarcts play an important role in pathogenesis, the resulting necrotic bone providing an excellent culture media for bacterial organisms which happen to settle there. While over 80% of hematogenous osteomyelitis in persons without a hemoglobinopathy is staphylococcal, the majority of cases seen in patients with sickle cell anemia (or S-C or S-Thalassemia) are caused by salmonella. However, cases of osteomyelitis due to pneumococcal and staphylococcal organisms are also observed. The basis for the increased susceptibility to systemic salmonella infection is not known. Although local infarcts have been postulated as rendering the gastrointestinal tract less capable of resisting invasion by enteric bacteria, there is no direct evidence to support such a theory.

Figure 46. Lobar pneumonia on x-ray. Blood and throat cultures grew *D. pneumoniae.* Also note cardiomegaly which is a common finding in sickle cell anemia.

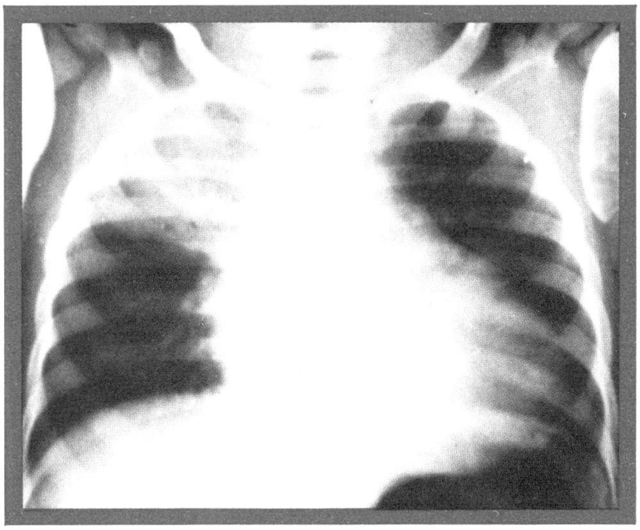

PULMONARY MANIFESTATIONS

Acute febrile pulmonary disease is the single most common reason for hospitalization of patients with sickle cell anemia, most of these acute episodes being bacterial pneumonia—lobar, (Fig. 46), segmental or bronchopneumonia. Pneumonia is probably at least 100 times as frequent in children with sickle cell anemia than in the general pediatric population. The pneumococcus is the most common organism involved, although often no specific etiologic agent is demonstrated. While lobar pneumonia in otherwise normal individuals usually resolves rapidly with lysis of fever within 48 hours after institution of appropriate antibiotic, there is much slower resolution in the patient with sickle cell anemia. Also the tendency to recurrent episodes is much greater in the latter. It has been postulated that regional hypoxia occurring in pneumonia increases sickling, thereby increasing viscosity, stasis and further ischemia. This may then complicate the resolution of the inflammatory process.

Pneumonia or Pulmonary Infarct?

Minute pulmonary infarcts probably occur repeatedly and go undetected clinically or radiographically. However in patients presenting with acute febrile pulmonary disease the differential diagnosis of pneumonia from pulmonary infarction may be difficult. The failure to obtain a bacteriologic diagnosis and the known propensity for pulmonary infarction which may resemble pneumonia both clinically and radiographically often lead to diagnostic uncertainty. Chest pain, splinting, rapid shallow respirations, fever, cough and wedge-shaped densities may be characteristic of both pneumonia and pulmonary infarction. A large infarct may be radiographically indistinguishable from segmental consolidation and/or atelectasis; and, to add to the confusion, it is known that secondary infection may be superimposed in the devitalized areas following infarction. Two additional diagnostic techniques which may occasionally be helpful are radioisotope scanning and angiography. The perfusion scan with ^{131}I MAA (macroaggregated human serum albumin labelled with ^{131}I) is the most widely used of the pulmonary radioisotope studies. It is a relatively simple procedure with no significant associated risk. By this method the distribution of pulmonary blood flow can be inferred from the distribution of radioactive particles deposited in the lung (Fig. 47). However, the appearance of the defect in the lung scan pattern that represents a pulmonary infarct is often not sufficiently characteristic to establish this diagnosis. Unfortunately, other parenchymal lesions of the lung, including lobar pneumonia, may result in a similar pattern of decreased radioactivity.

Selective pulmonary angiography may be of greater diagnostic help, especially in the case of a large pulmonary infarct. In such cases angiography may demonstrate an abrupt interruption of blood flow. However angiography does not always resolve the problem either, as hypoperfusion does not always indicate infarction. For example, in segmental atelectasis reactive vasospasm may result in poor perfusion. Also one must be aware that the hyperosmotic contrast agents used for angiography may promote intravascular sickling. This risk is minimized by transfusing the patient with packed cells pre-angiography and careful maintenance of adequate hydration before, during and after the procedure. However, unless treatment differs because a pulmonary infarct is demonstrated, angiography should not be done.

As a result of repeated small infarcts and scarring, the lungs of adolescents and adults with sickle cell anemia may be less radiolucent than normal. Occasionally pulmonary arterial changes (intimal proliferation) and/or severe scarring in the lungs may result in cor pulmonale.

CARDIOVASCULAR MANIFESTATIONS

Cardiovascular manifestations frequently result from the following: (1) chronic anemia, (2) pulmonary arterial occlusions leading to cor pulmonale, and (3) myocardial damage resulting from small infarcts as well as iron deposition.

In children cardiac abnormalities consist of cardiomegaly and tachycardia, usually associated with exertional dyspnea and a "hemic murmur." The

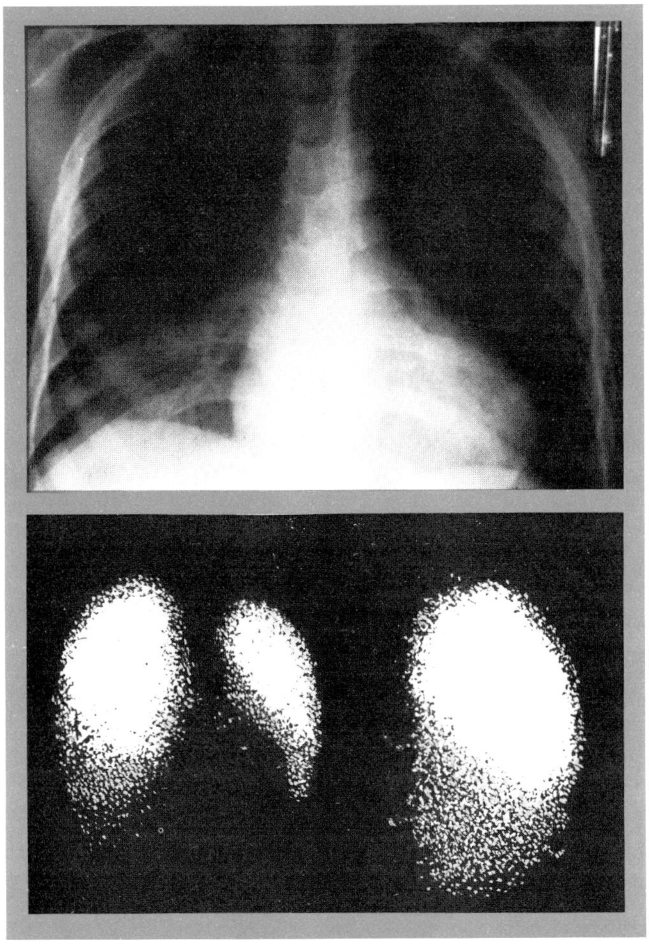

A

B

Figure 47. Pulmonary infarct vs pneumonia.
A. Chest x-ray shows right lower lobe consolidation.
B. Anterior and R. lateral lung scans demonstrate a perfusion defect at right base anterolaterally.

latter is a blowing systolic murmur over the mitral or pulmonic areas but which may be heard over any part of the precordium. This murmur results from increased pulmonary blood flow (relative pulmonic stenosis). In patients with severe anemia a diastolic murmur may also be heard. This probably reflects relative tricuspid or mitral stenosis resulting from the greatly increased blood flow. Another characteristic feature is accentuation of the pulmonic closure sound, with fixed splitting of the second sound. Roentgenograms reveal some degree of cardiomegaly (both left and right ventricles are enlarged) and increased pulmonary markings.

Several additional factors contribute to the progressive cardiac decompensation seen in adolescents or adults. Arteriovenous shunts have been demonstrated in the pulmonary as well as peripheral circulation. This pulmonary shunting results in decreased arterial oxygen saturation. Repeated small infarcts, fibrosis and hemosiderosis further impair myocardial function. Occlusion of small pulmonary arteries may result in pulmonary hypertension and chronic cor pulmonale. In the older patient congestive heart failure is common and may be intractible.

Sickle cell anemia may mimic rheumatic fever, making diagnosis of the latter difficult in a patient known to have sickle cell disease. Fever, migratory joint pain with swelling, cardiac murmurs and even pericarditis may occur in either. Electrocardiographic abnormalities are also frequent in sickle cell anemia. Although there is no characteristic ECG pattern, P-R interval prolongation and nonspecific ST segment and T wave changes are common.

The sedimentation rate may be slow in sickle cell anemia even in the presence of active rheumatic fever, and therefore one must rely on other diagnostic criteria. A therapeutic trial of salicylates may be helpful—dramatic response being indicative of rheumatic fever.

SKELETAL MANIFESTATIONS

Bone and Joint Infarcts. Severe pain occurs with bone infarcts in any area. Certain sites are more commonly involved. While dactylitis predominates in young children, in adults the head of the femur and humerus are particularly prone to develop infarcts as the vessels supplying these sites are long and tortuous and collateral circulation is poor. The

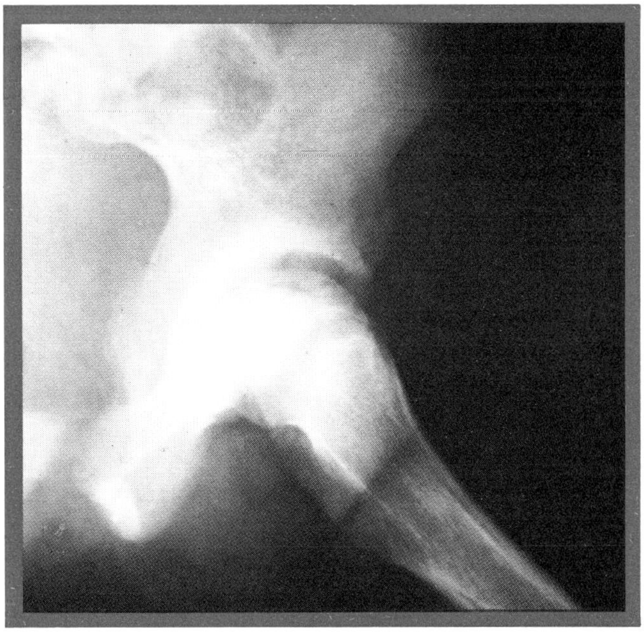

Figure 48. Aseptic necrosis with collapse of the femoral head in 17 year old girl with S-C hemoglobinopathy.

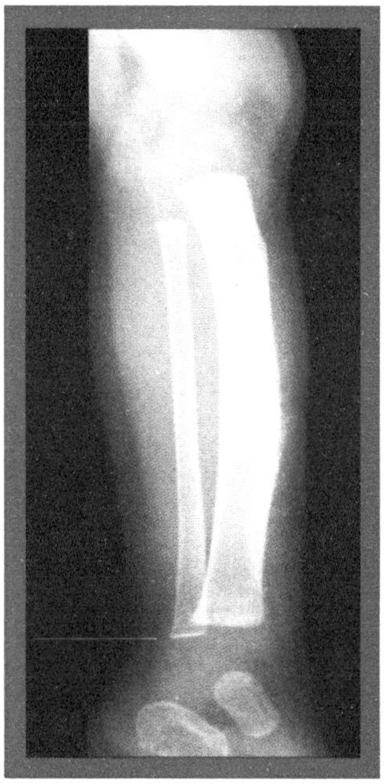

Figure 50. Bone changes resulting from infarction. Note rarefaction, subperiosteal new bone formation and periosteal elevation.

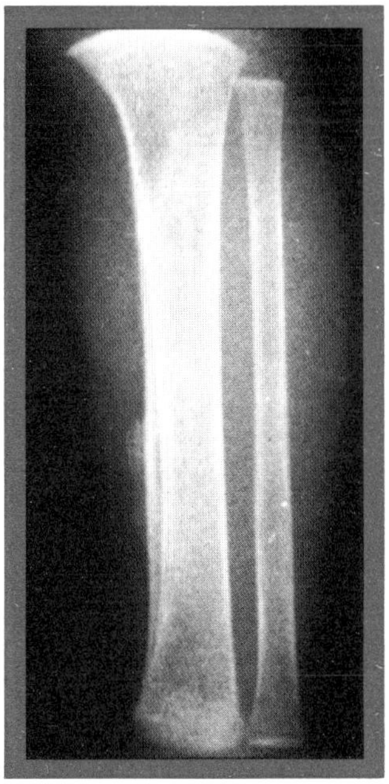

Figure 51. Similar abnormalities in another child, resulting from tibial infarcts.

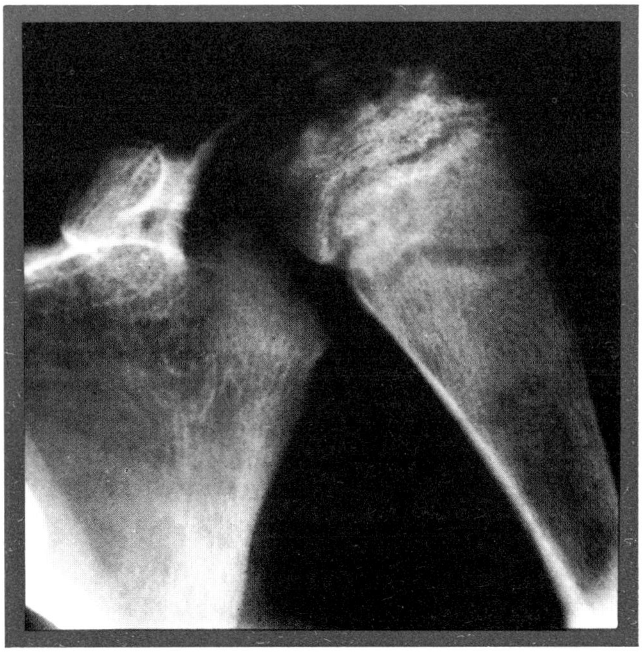

Figure 49. Aseptic necrosis of humeral head in 13 year old boy with sickle cell anemia.

lesions produced by vascular occlusion due to sickled cells have a roentgenologic appearance similar to those seen in other avascular lesions such as Legge-Calve-Perthes disease. It is interesting to note that avascular necrosis of the femoral head is not seen in young children with sickle cell disease as the artery in the ligamentum teres is patent, providing a dual blood supply to the femoral head. Also the arteries through the hip capsule are short and of large calibre.

Interruption of blood supply usually leads to the following sequence of events: (1) necrosis of bone, (2) repair, characterized by revascularization, re-ossification, and the resorption of dead bone. If revascularization does not take place degenerative changes in the cartilage and synovial membrane occur, the joint space becomes narrow, the smooth synovial surface becomes jagged and irregular, and the femoral head fragments and collapses (Fig. 48).

Varying degrees of pain and disability often result from this destructive process.

Juxta-articular infarction may also occur in the humeral head (Fig. 49). Although collapse of the humeral head may eventually occur, it is much less common in this non-weight bearing joint as compared to collapse of the femoral head. Pain and disability are also generally less in the former.

Other commonly affected bones are the tibia (Figs. 50, 51) and fibula. Acute infarction is associated with severe pain, localized tenderness and swelling. Early lesions show no x-ray changes but later roentgenographic findings may be strikingly similar to those of osteomyelitis, with radiolucent areas (rarefaction reflecting resorption of dead trabeculae) and subperiosteal new bone formation. To add to the diagnostic confusion, it is known that bacterial osteomyelitis may be superimposed on an infarct of bone, the devitalized tissue serving as an excellent culture medium for bacterial growth.

Skull and Long Bones. The bone marrow in sickle cell anemia is hypercellular, containing little fat. In older children the red marrow recedes from the tubular bones of the hands and feet, but in contrast with normals, remains in the small bones of the ankles, wrists and shafts of long bones. As a consequence of marrow hyperplasia there is widening of the medullary cavities and thinning of trabeculae and cortex. These changes are observed in the skull, vertebrae, and long bones, and are much more commonly seen in adolescents and adults than in young children. The cranial vault may show widening of the diploic space with thinning of the outer table (Fig. 52). This is more prominent in the frontal and parietal regions. The diploe itself may be coarsely granular in texture; (ground glass appearance). Occasionally, trabeculae may arrange themselves radially resulting in a "hair on end" or "porcupine quill" appearance (Fig. 52B). Although seen in a small percentage of patients with sickle cell anemia, the latter is more commonly seen in thalassemia major.

Figure 52. Characteristic skull changes (in identical twins with sickle cell anemia) resulting from marrow hyperplasia **A.** widening of diploic space with thinning of outer table. **B.** "hair on end" appearance more characteristic of thalassemia major, but occasionally seen in sickle cell anemia.

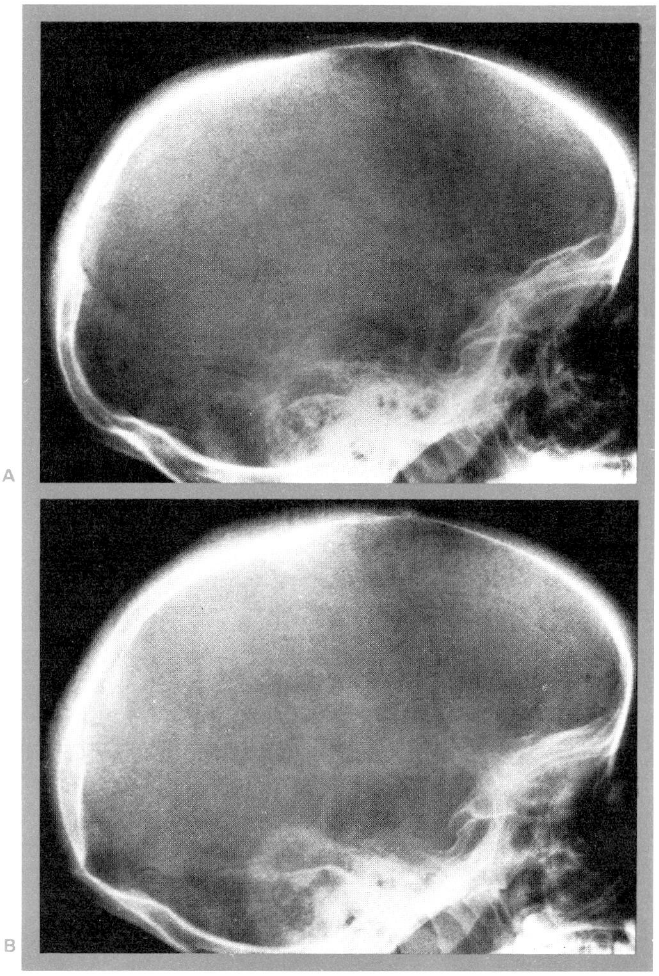

Spine Changes. In adolescents and young adults there may be osteoporosis of the vertebrae with coarsened trabeculae. Vertebral bodies are characteristically flattened, with an increase in width and decrease in height. There may be biconvexity of the disc spaces, producing the so-called "fish mouth

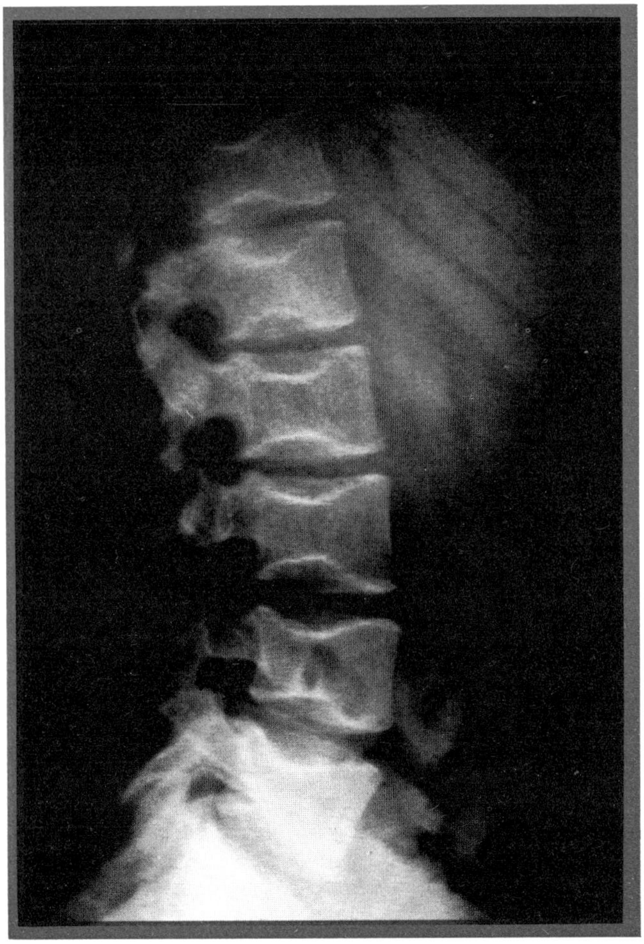

Figure 53. "Fish mouth vertebrae" in 16 year old girl with sickle cell anemia.

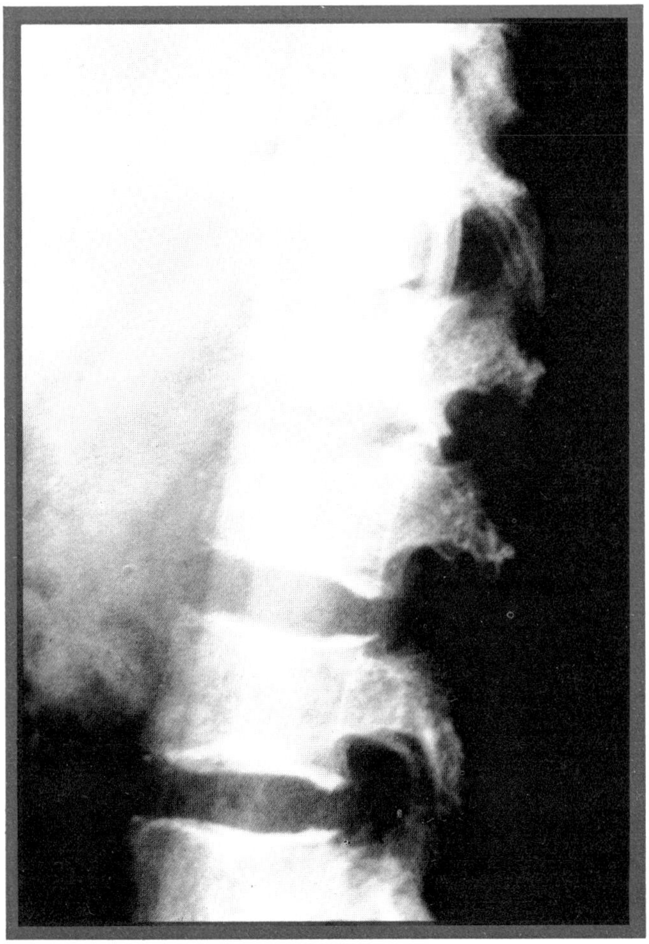

Figure 54. "Fish mouth vertebrae" in 18 year old girl with sickle cell anemia. Note destructive changes in lower thoracic and lumbar spine with collapsed vertebral body LI and compression of L2.

vertebra" sign (Fig. 53). The biconcavity of the vertebral bodies probably reflects several factors: (1) weight-bearing by bones which are structurally weak and actively proliferating, (2) central infarcts with growth arrest in the central sclerotic area and more rapid marginal bone growth. These changes occur only during the growing period, stopping after epiphyseal union. Osteoporosis, destruction and collapse of the weakened vertebral bodies (Fig. 54) may also cause compression deformities.

Other Skeletal Changes. From approximately 7 years of age there is x-ray evidence of marrow hyperplasia in the ribs, with broadening of individual ribs (Fig. 40). The iliac bones show a characteristic coarse trabecular pattern, and often there are irregular stippled calcific densities which presumably result from marrow infarcts.

Skeletal Maturation and Stature. Adolescents with sickle cell anemia often weigh less and have a relative delay in skeletal maturation. Height varies, but it is generally less than that of controls in early teens. By late teenage, however, the average height is as great as that of non-sicklers. This greater than normal increase in stature during adolescence has been interpreted by some as reflecting the delay in skeletal maturation.

LEG ULCERS

Although rarely seen in children, leg ulcers are a common cause of morbidity in adults with sickle cell anemia. Ulcerations most often occur over the malleoli (Fig. 55) and appear as rounded, punched out lesions with a dirty-gray base (rather than healthy granulation tissue) and undermined edges. While slight trauma is often the inciting event, these ulcerations result from stasis in small blood vessels—arteries, capillaries and venules—often with obliterative vascular changes. In some patients the ulcers become massive, encircling the leg. Healing is quite slow, and there is a tendency to recurrence. Cellulitis, lymphangitis, bacteremia and thrombosis are common complications.

RENAL LESION

Functional and anatomic renal lesions appear to occur regularly in sickle cell disease. These occur as a consequence of sickling in the vasa recta of the renal medulla. There is gradual obliteration of the vasa recta, leading to a concentrating defect as these vessels form an intrinsic part of the countercurrent multiplication system of the long loops of Henle. The collecting ducts, medullary structures dependent on the vasa recta for their blood supply, may also develop functional abnormalities. Thus, so-called "sickle cell nephropathy" is characterized by defective renal concentration and acidification, despite an increased glomerular filtration rate.

The juxta-medullary nephrons (14% of total neph-

Figure 55. Leg ulcers in 2 young adults with sickle cell anemia.

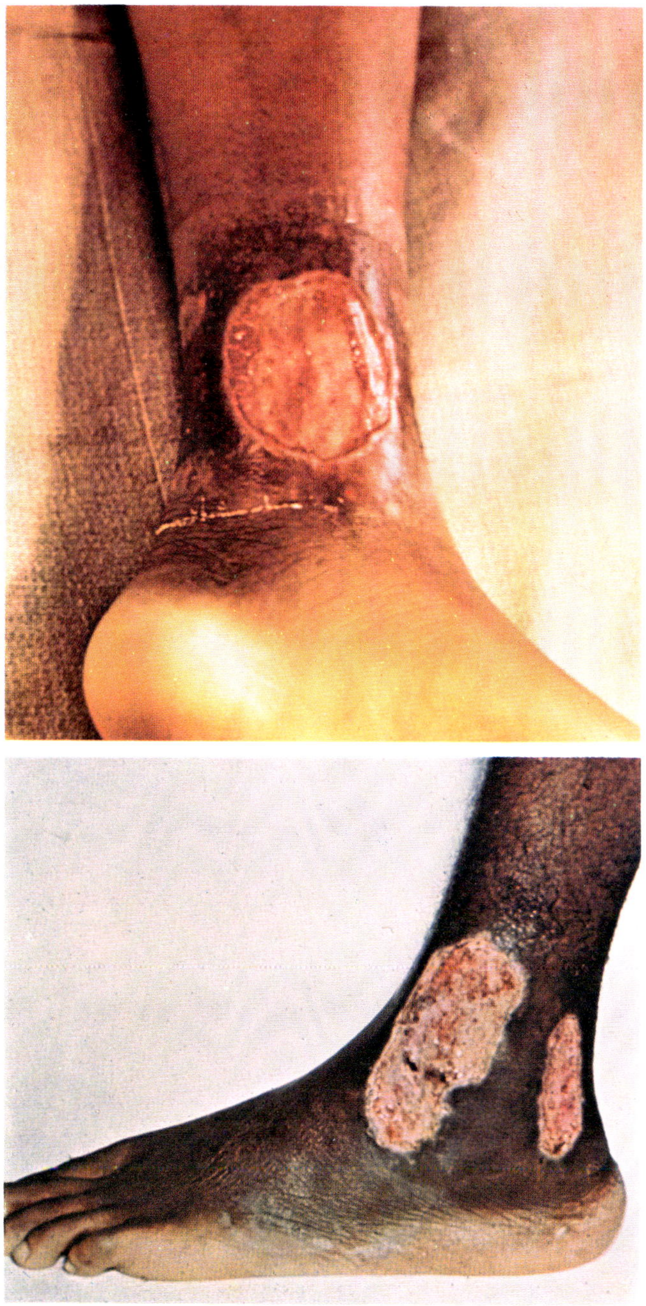

Figure 56. Diagram of a juxtamedullary nephron and its vasa recta. Obstruction of the latter ultimately results in renal concentrating defect.

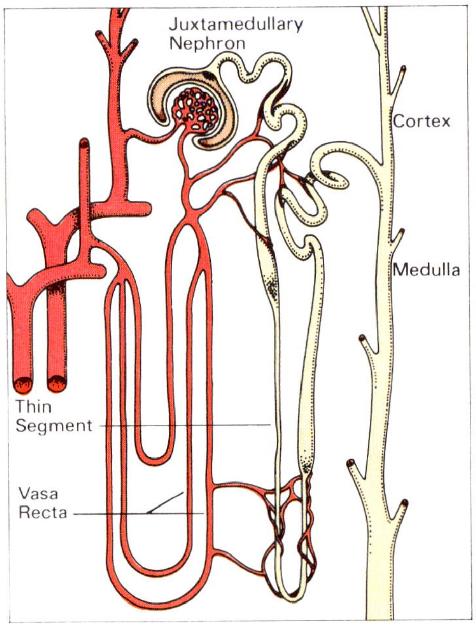

Figure 57. Microradioangiograph of a pyramid from **A.** a normal kidney (72 years), **B.** sickle cell anemia kidney (31 years), and **C.** sickle cell hemoglobin C disease kidney (5 years).

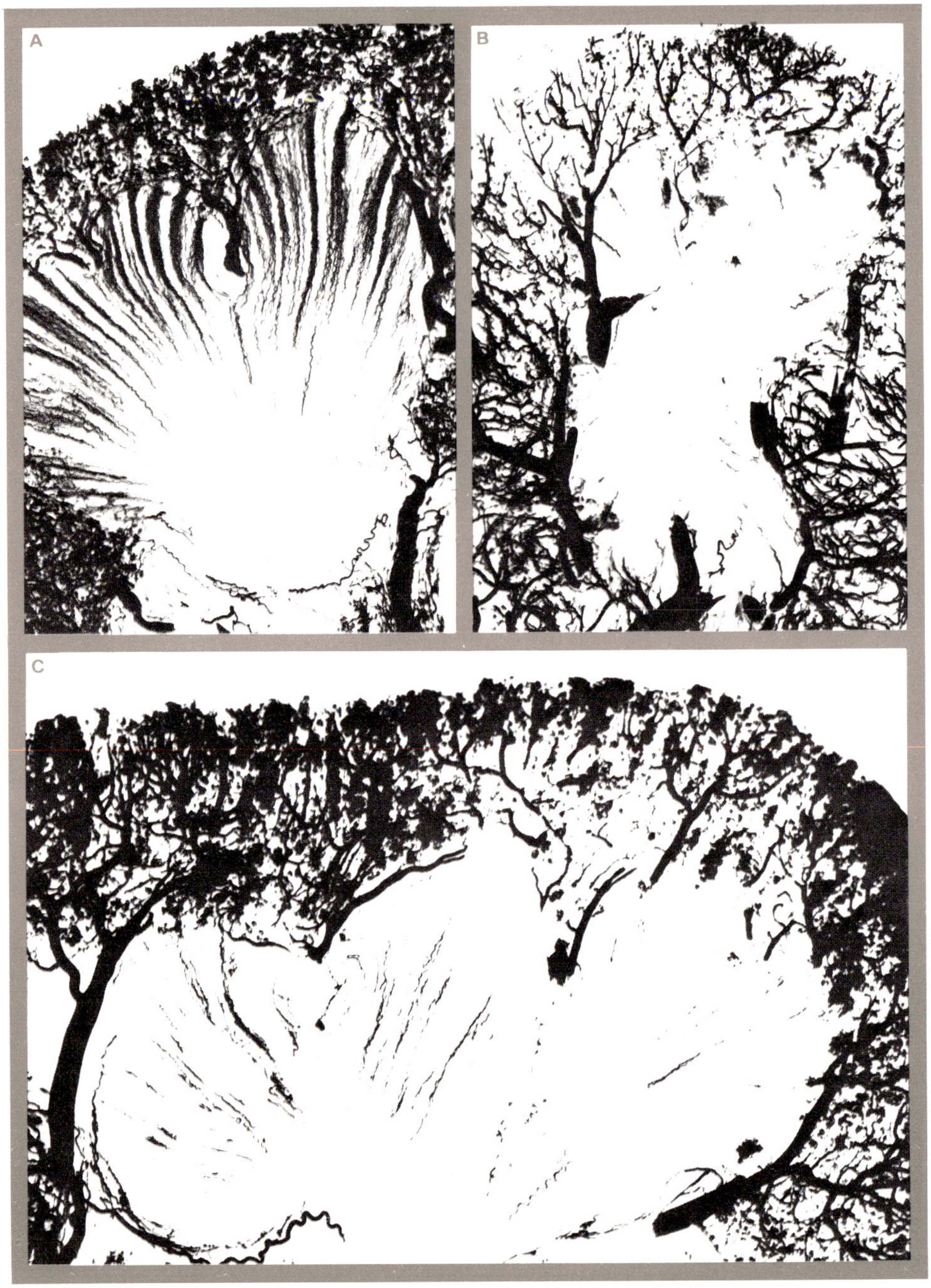

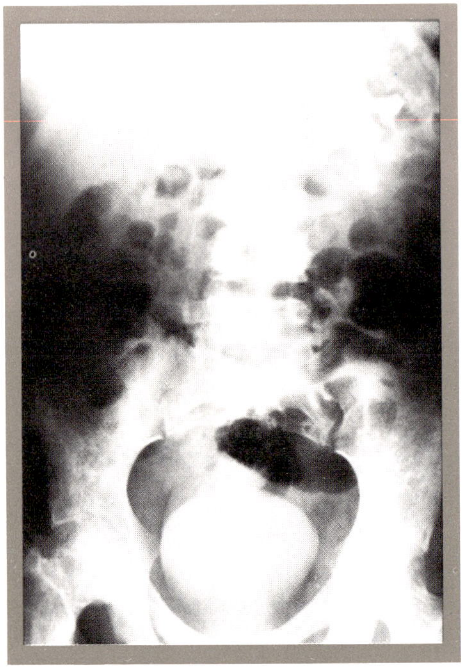

Figure 58. Pyelocaliectasis involving left kidney in 18 year old girl with sickle cell anemia. Note dilatation of renal pelvis and blunting of calyces.

ron population) with their long loops of Henle extending into the inner medullary zone and renal papilla (Fig. 56) are responsible for increases in osmolarity (up to 1200 m Osm) during thirsting. If the functioning of the long loops of Henle and vasa recta is disturbed, concentrating capacity is reduced. It has been postulated that hemoglobin S erythrocytes traversing the normally hyperosmotic medulla during hydropenia undergo sickling. The resulting increased viscosity and stasis promote hypoxia and acidosis, further sickling and vaso-occlusion. While collaterals may develop, these will lack the highly specialized spatial configuration of the vasa recta, parallel to the long loops of Henle necessary for countercurrent multiplication. Microradio-angiographic studies (Fig. 57) have demonstrated gross lesions of the renal medulla, with almost complete absence of vasa recta. The few remaining are dilated and end blindly, suggesting obliteration. At a later age and to a lesser degree, one may see similar changes in SC disease and sickle trait. In SC and AS kidneys there is a gradual loss of vasa recta and loss of normal bundle architecture (Fig. 57 B & C).

In persons with sickle cell anemia under 10 years of age the hyposthenuria is variable and appears to be reversible by multiple transfusions (transfused RBC probably slowly replace the stagnant SS erythrocytes in the vasa recta, restoring normal circulation). Over 10 years of age concentrating capacity is reduced to a very narrow range and is not reversible by transfusion. This fixation of concentrating power at 400-500 milliosmoles does not occur until much later in those with SC or AS hemoglobin.

Papillary renal necrosis, resulting from sickling and occlusion of terminal arterioles and capillaries may be manifest by unilateral hematuria. Such changes may be seen in persons with SC disease or sickle trait. Using standard radiographic techniques

Figure 59. Nine year old boy with hemiparesis and muscle atrophy (left arm and left leg) following CNS infarction.

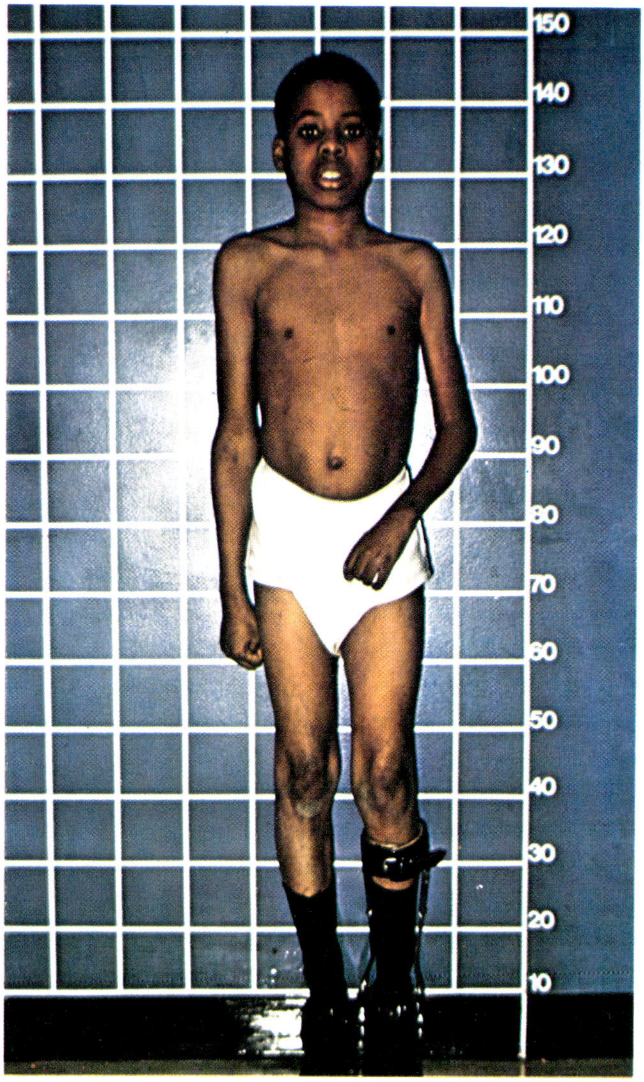

(intravenous pyelography), filling defects and papillary necrosis are the most frequently observed renal changes. Calyceal blunting ("sickle cell caliectasis") probably results from congestion, necrosis and fibrosis (Fig. 58).

There is also an increased incidence of urinary

tract infection, particularly pyelonephritis, in older children and adults with sickle cell disease. Scarring of the renal medulla and structural abnormalities predisposing to focal collection of urine no doubt enhance urinary tract infection in these individuals.

NEUROLOGICAL MANIFESTATIONS

Neurological manifestations are frequent, although the exact incidence is unknown. While neurologic dysfunction may be related to meningitis, or such coincidental conditions as berry aneurysm, eclampsia in pregnancy, subdural hematoma or tuberculoma, it most often results from vaso-occlusion and infarction. Vaso-occlusion by sickled cells may occur in any part of the nervous system. The onset of symptoms is often sudden, with focal or generalized convulsions, hemiparesis, aphasia and coma. Occasionally attacks may be transient and reversible, but all too often they are irreversible, resulting in severe neurologic sequelae (Fig. 59) or even death. Episodes of CNS infarction tend to be recurrent—the individual with sickle cell anemia who has had one or more CNS infarcts is more likely to have recurrent ones than a patient who has not had prior CNS involvement. No doubt an already compromised circulation plays a role in the greater tendency to such recurrences. Spastic quadriplegia and severe disability may be the unfortunate end result.

While it was previously held that CNS manifestations in sickle cell anemia resulted exclusively from small vessel obstruction, angiographic studies (Figs. 60 and 61 have indicated that this is not the case. The majority of patients studied by arteriography have had partial or complete occlusion of such major intracranial vessels as the internal carotid, middle and anterior cerebral arteries. The process of occlusion of these major vessels appears to be a progressive disorder. Occlusion of the vasa vasorum (nutrient arteries) may result in ischemia of the walls of larger arteries, which then leads to intimal and medial wall proliferation. The latter may eventually result in obstruction of blood flow through the larger vessel.

Common neurologic manifestations include headache, hemiplegia, aphasia, convulsions, nystagmus, pupillary changes, blindness and paresthesias. Such symptoms most often result from CNS infarction, but massive subarachnoid hemorrhage may also occur. This too may result from local damage to a vessel wall following vaso-occlusion and infarction. While relatively uncommon, subarachnoid hemorrhage is associated with a high mortality rate. Some feel that it should be investigated by angiography whenever possible, as an operable congenital aneurysm might be disclosed. However, the patient may be too critically ill to tolerate such a procedure. Whenever angiography is done it should be preceded by transfusions with packed cells to reduce the percentage of hemoglobin S RBC, as the hypertonic contrast material used is capable of inducing sickling. Also, the patient should be well hydrated and the volume and concentration of contrast material to be injected should be minimized to permit adequate visualization without undue risk of intravascular sickling.

Retinopathy. A variety of ophthalmologic abnormalities may occur in sickle cell disease. As elsewhere in the body these changes result from sickling, stasis and occlusion of small blood vessels. The high rate of glycolysis in the retina no doubt predisposes to rapid depletion of oxygen from the RBC, and the presence of an end-arteriole system in the retina further predisposes to anoxia and tissue damage once occlusion occurs. The end result may be decreased visual acuity or even blindness.

The characteristic retinal changes in sickle cell anemia as observed by indirect ophthalmoscopy are circular, black chorioretinal scars. These so-called

Figure 60. Partial obstruction of superior saggital sinus as demonstrated by cerebral angiography. Note collateral vessel. Arrows indicate portion of vessel occluded. The patient, a 10 year old boy, presented with severe headaches.

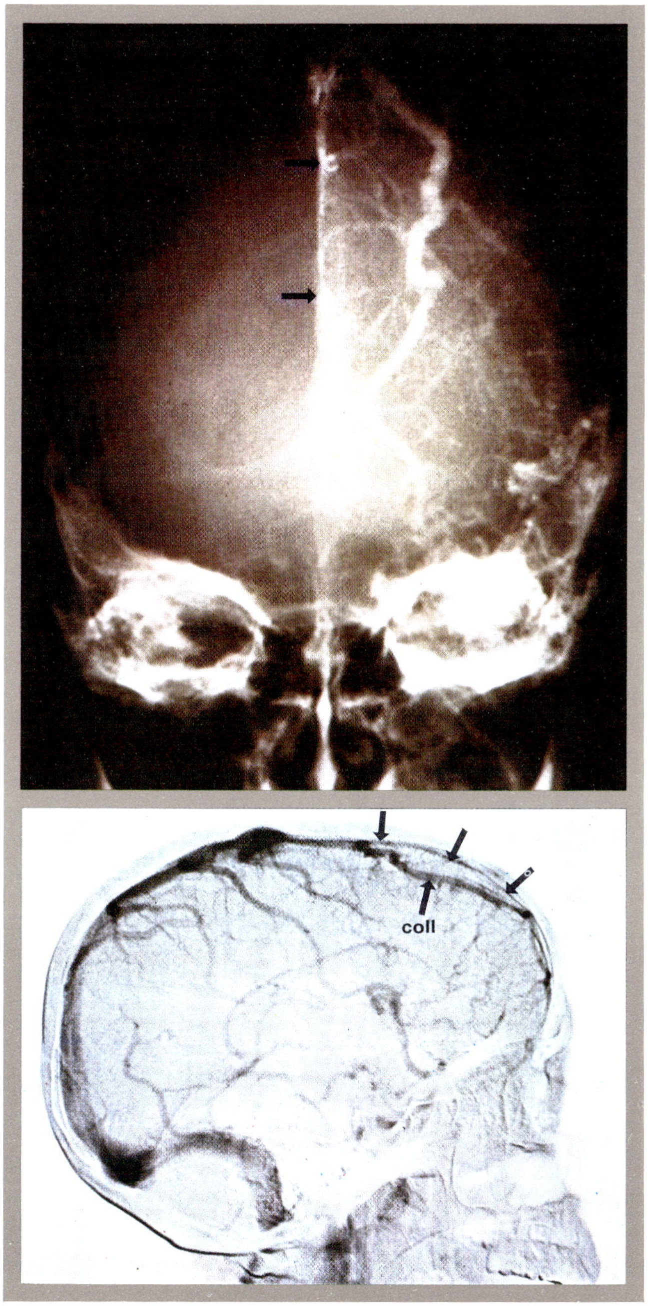

Figure 61. A. Occlusion of 4th opercular branch of R. middle cerebral artery as demonstrated by cerebral angiography. This 4 year old child presented with focal convulsions followed by hemiparesis. **B.** Arrows show small microaneurysms coming from temporal branch of R. middle cerebral artery. The study also demonstrates increased blood supply to ganglionic branches of right temporal lobe.

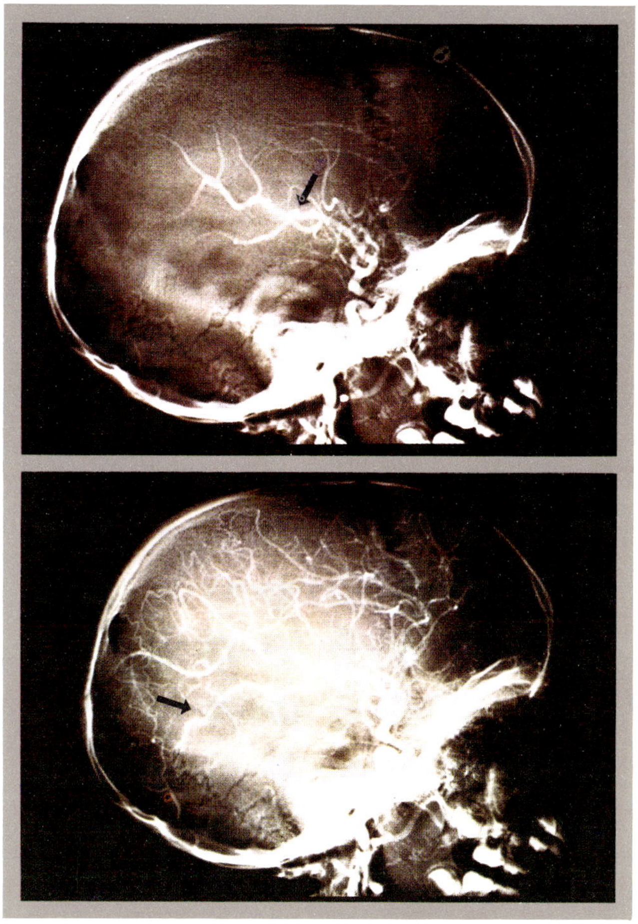

A

B

"black sunbursts" probably result from small infarcts or hemorrhages. Their presence does not ordinarily affect visual acuity.

Proliferative retinopathy is seen in young adults with sickle cell anemia, but is much more common in those with SC disease or S-Thalassemia. Clinically symptomatic and significant stages of proliferative sickle retinopathy (PSR) are frequently observed in individuals with SC disease over 20 years of age. The sequence of events in the pathogenesis of PSR consists of sickling, stasis and peripheral arteriolar occlusion in the retina, the formation of arteriovenous anastomoses, and neovascular proliferation. Leakage of blood from these neovascularizations may result in vitreous hemorrhages and retinal detachment. Loss of vision may result. By the technique of fluorescein angiography (Fig. 62) tufts of newly proliferating vessels resembling "sea fans" are most often seen in the superotemporal quadrant of the retina. One can also see leakage of dye from these lesions into the vitreous.

Figure 62. Proliferative sickle retinopathy. Neovascular lesions ("sea fans") demonstrated by fluorescein angiography.

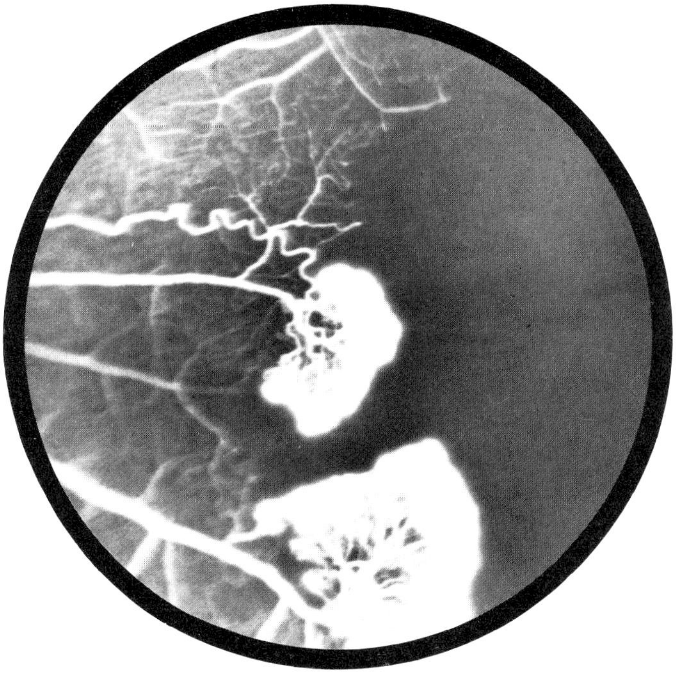

REPRODUCTIVE SYSTEM

Individuals with sickle cell anemia have hypogonadism and delayed development of secondary sexual characteristics. In females there is a delay in estrogen stimulation, manifest by delayed onset of menarche and decreased fertility.

Pregnancy. The apparent decreased fertility no doubt also reflects infrequent intercourse, because of chronic illness or even death before childbearing becomes a reasonable possibility. In those who do become pregnant, problems may arise, especially during late pregnancy, parturition and the puerperium. The demands of an expanding vascular bed and blood volume, as well as an accelerating metabolic drain by the fetus in an already chronically ill patient may result in a worsening of her status. One complication rather frequently observed is that of an increasing anemia, probably reflecting folic acid deficiency. In addition, the incidence of such complications as congestive heart failure, pulmonary infarction, pyelonephritis and toxemia is reportedly increased. In other respects, however, the pregnant patient with sickle cell anemia appears to do as well as when not pregnant. The frequency and severity of crises during pregnancy is probably unaltered from patterns expressed prior to pregnancy.

Fetal Salvage. Fetal salvage, defined as the ratio of surviving infants to the number of pregnancies, is notably depressed in sickle cell anemia (55-60%, in contrast to 87% in normal populations). This poor salvage rate reflects an increased incidence of spontaneous abortions (20%), stillbirths and neonatal deaths (14%). The incidence of prematurity and premature labor is also increased (20-25%). Intrauterine hypoxia caused by sickling, stasis and occlusion involving uterine and decidual arteries has been casually implicated; however, such factors as chronic anemia, maternal debility and the high incidence of toxemia may be involved as well.

In summary, pregnancy in sickle cell anemia results in smaller babies, greater numbers of premature deaths and abortions, and a higher incidence of pulmonary and renal complications, toxemia and congestive heart failure than is observed in the general population. While opinion varies considerably concerning the overall effects of pregnancy, most observations suggest that the frequency and severity of crises is unaltered from previous patterns.

Priapism. A small but significant percentage of boys with sickle cell anemia will suffer priapism, a persistent painful erection of the penis. This condition can occur at any age and may persist for hours, days or even weeks. While the pathogenesis is not entirely clear, it is thought that sluggish blood flow in the corpora cavernosa and lowered oxygen tension lead to sickling, stasis and occlusion of venous return. A vicious cycle ensues, with venous occlusion resulting in more stasis, hypoxia and sickling. Prolonged episodes of priapism, with or without surgical intervention (see section on treatment) may result in impotence.

LIFE EXPECTANCY AND CAUSES OF DEATH

The clinical picture of sickle cell anemia is quite variable, some having relatively little symptomatology while others may die or become severely disabled early in life. The majority are plagued with intermittent pain crises, bacterial infections and easy fatigability resulting from chronic anemia, and have slowly progressive deterioration of various tissues and organs resulting from repeated infarcts. It has been estimated by some that approximately 50% of patients die before the age of 20 years and most do not survive beyond 40. However, statistical data is conspicuously lacking and these figures may not be accurate. A disproportionate number of deaths occur in infancy or early childhood, usually as the result of overwhelming bacterial infections or suddenly developing severe anemia *(splenic sequestration crisis)*. In one reported series 10 of 64 children diagnosed in the first year of life as having sickle cell anemia died before 12 months of age; in 8 of the 10 the cause of death was overwhelming bacterial infection. In another series of 207 children between the ages of 2 and 14 years who were followed for a 5 year period there were 19 deaths, 13 of which occurred in children under 6 years of age. Most deaths resulted from a sudden catastrophic event—overwhelming infection, acute splenic sequestration crisis or acute cerebrovascular occlusion. Thus while rigorous attention to health care is strongly recommended for all with sickle cell anemia, it would appear that some of these deaths would not be prevented by such means. Until an effective means of preventing intravascular sickling is found, these catastrophic events will no doubt continue. In our own experience at the Children's Hospital of Michigan 16 children died within a 6 year period; of these, 9 were under 3 years of age. The same three causes of death predominated—namely overwhelming bacterial infection, splenic sequestration and CNS infarction. In another group of 166 children and adults followed for 11 years there were 15 deaths, 9 in children under 4 years of age. While the risk of bacterial infection is markedly reduced after age three years, in those dying in adolescense or adulthood, bacterial infection is still the commonest cause of death. Other causes include cerebrovascular accidents (infarction and/or CNS hemorrhage), chronic renal failure, cardiac failure and hepatic disease. In the tropics, parasitic diseases are frequent terminal complications.

Clinical Picture of Sickle Trait

It is estimated that 8-10% of American Blacks have sickle cell trait. The incidence is much higher in certain parts of Africa, reportedly being 30-45% in some East African Bantu tribes, and 20-30% in West Africa as a whole. Those who are heterozygous for the sickle cell gene appear to have a selective advantage in regions where malaria is common, as the sickle trait appears to afford some protection against infection with Plasmodium falciparum (see p. 68).

Persons with sickle cell trait are not anemic, have no physical abnormalities, are usually asymptomatic and have a normal life span. The trait can be demonstrated *in vitro* by a variety of laboratory techniques based on the ability of the RBC to sickle when oxygen tension is lowered. As determined by electrophoresis, hemoglobin S constitutes 20-45% of the total hemoglobin, the remainder (55-80%) being hemoglobin A. Hemoglobin F is present in normal amounts (less than 2% after 1 year of age). Values for hemoglobin, hematocrit, RBC indices and reticulocyte count are normal and on examination of the peripheral blood smear RBC appear normochromic and normocytic. RBC survival time is also normal.

While individuals with the trait are generally asymptomatic under normal physiologic conditions, intravascular sickling, vaso-occlusion and infarction can occur if oxygen tension is sufficiently lowered. Indeed sickle cell trait can, under certain extreme circumstances, be fatal. Hypoventilation during general anesthesia is a potentially fatal hazard which must be avoided. Splenic infarction has been reported in AS subjects during high altitude flying in unpressurized aircraft (over 10,000 feet) and during periods of vigorous exercise at high altitudes. In the latter instance, the combination of hypoxia, acidosis, excess lactate and high blood viscosity from dehydration no doubt enhances intravascular sickling. However, air travel should not be regarded as hazardous as modern aircraft maintain cabin atmospheric pressures equivalent to altitudes of 7,000 feet.

Gross hematuria, renal infarction and renal papillary necrosis may also be seen on occasion in sickle trait. A gradual and progressive loss of renal concentrating (and acidifying) capacity is regularly observed in adults with sickle cell trait, a fixed maximum of 400-450 milliosmoles being reached around 60 years of age. Microradioangiographic studies in adult sickle trait kidneys reveal a reduced number of vasa recta and spiralling and dilatation of the remaining ones. These medullary changes are intermediate between the pattern seen in individuals with sickle cell anemia and normals (see p. 51).

Sickle cell trait is more than an interesting genetic anomaly without clinical significance. Under certain circumstances, albeit unphysiological ones, severe disability or even death may occur as a result. Fortunately such severe complications are rare, but one should be aware of the potential for intravascular sickling in these individuals.

While the incidence of pyelonephritis during pregnancy is somewhat increased in AS individuals, fertility, pregnancy and delivery are normal. There is no increase in the incidence of spontaneous abortion, prematurity, stillbirths or neonatal deaths as seen in sickle cell anemia.

Hemoglobin Variant Combinations

Selected hemoglobinopathies (Hb C, Hb D, Hb O) and other hemoglobin variants (Hb F, Thalassemia) resulting from abnormal rates of hemoglobin chain synthesis are briefly considered because of occasional coexistence and interaction with Hb S. The severity of the clinical syndromes in these doubly heterozygous states in general correlates well with the physicochemical properties of the hemoglobin mixtures. Knowledge of these states should have value in genetic counselling.

HEMOGLOBIN C

This abnormal hemoglobin results from the substitution of a single amino acid, lysine for glutamic acid, in the same position that the Hb S abnormality occurs. A brief description of Hb C trait and homozygous Hb C disease follows, as a basis for later comparison with the doubly heterozygous state, SC hemoglobinopathy. Although not a standard laboratory procedure, in all 3 states crystal forms of Hb C can be induced and demonstrated by mixing peripheral blood with hypertonic saline (Fig. 63).

Hemoglobin C (Georgetown) and C (Harlem) are rare sickling hemoglobins which have the same electrophoretic mobility as the common C hemoglobin. The amino acid substitutions are different, however, and affected individuals reported have been asymptomatic.

Hemoglobin C Trait (AC). It is estimated that 2% of American Blacks possess one gene for C hemoglobin. The highest carrier rates (20%) have been found in Northern Ghana (West Africa). Individuals with C trait (AC) are asymptomatic and have normal hemoglobin values and reticulocyte counts, normal RBC indices and normal (or near normal) RBC survival times. There are no characteristic physical abnormalities. Examination of the peripheral blood film reveals 5-40% target cells, but no other distinguishing morphologic features. On electrophoresis (Fig. 64) there is a band of A hemoglobin (constituting 60-75% of the total hemoglobin) and a smaller band of C hemoglobin (25-40%).

Homozygous Hemoglobin C (CC). The homozygous state is uncommon (estimated incidence 1/6,000 American Blacks). Most affected individuals have a mild hemolytic anemia although some have no anemia. Hemoglobin values vary between 9 and 14 gms % and reticulocyte counts are usually slightly elevated (1-7%). On electrophoresis there is a single, slow

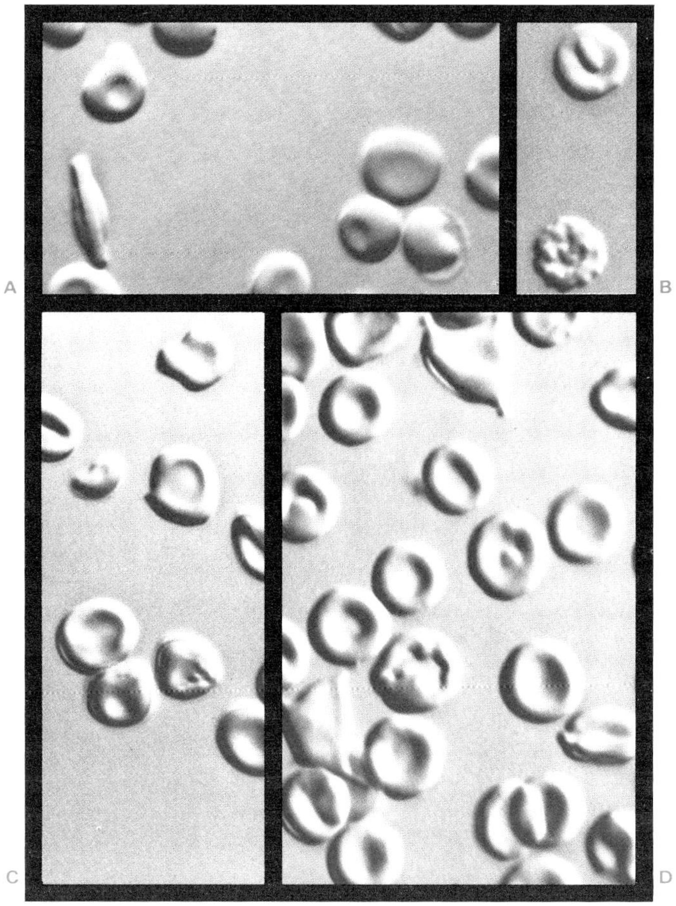

Figure 63. Nomarski micrographs of crystal formation on exposure to hypertonic Na Cl. These preparations were incubated at room temperature for 3 hours.
A. and B. From 2 different Hb CC subjects. C. From a Hb AC individual. D. From an individual with SC disease. Note resemblance of 2 cells to target cells. (X 2050).

moving band of hemoglobin quite near the origin. The most striking feature on examination of the peripheral blood smear is a large number of target cells (Fig. 65). Target cells are more numerous in dried smears made on a glass surface than when plasma-suspended cells are examined, 50-90% of RBC appearing as target cells in the former. The central density probably results from centrally located Hb C crystals, as well as membranous folds near the center of the cell. Some of the microcrystals may be pitted out by the reticuloendothelial elements of the spleen, with some loss of membrane. The latter probably accounts for the microspherocytes, which are also a characteristic feature in homozygous C disease.

Most affected individuals have a moderately enlarged spleen. Hepatomegaly is a variable finding. While some have recurrent episodes of arthralgia and/or abdominal pain, the majority are asymptomatic. There is no renal concentrating defect and growth and development as well as life span are generally normal.

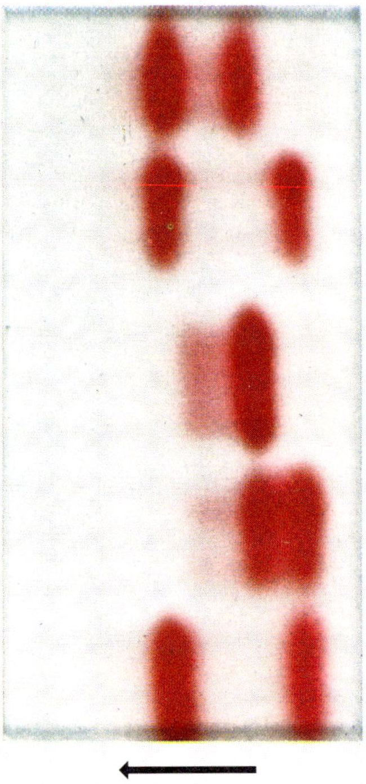

Figure 64. Hemoglobin electrophoresis on cellulose acetate.

S-C Hemoglobinopathy (Hemoglobin SC Disease). Although accurate statistics are not available, it is estimated that 1 in 1500 American Negroes have S-C hemoglobinopathy. This doubly heterozygous state is approximately 1/3 as common as sickle cell anemia. The incidence is considerably higher in certain parts of West Africa.

The clinical manifestations resulting from intravascular sickling and vaso-occlusion are generally less severe than those in individuals with sickle cell anemia but are extremely variable. Some affected individuals are asymptomatic, while others are severely disabled. The primary pathologic changes are referable to the presence of S hemoglobin.

The onset of symptoms occurs later in life than in sickle cell anemia, and some may indeed never have them. Approximately 50% have symptoms before 10 years of age, arthralgia, musculoskeletal and abdominal pains being the most common. These painful crises are less frequent and less severe than those seen in sickle cell anemia.

SC disease is characterized by a chronic hemolytic anemia of moderate degree, hemoglobin values ranging from 8-10 gms %. In most affected individuals the reticulocyte count is elevated (range 1-15%) and there is erythroid hyperplasia in the marrow. Characteristic features on peripheral blood smear include numerous target cells (40-80% of RBC), slight aniso- and poikilocytosis with occasional sickle forms and some polychromatophilic RBC (Fig. 66). Red cell survival, according to ^{51}Cr data, is shortened, T-1/2 being approximately 15 days. The resulting increase in bili-

Figure 65. Peripheral blood film from individual with homozygous C hemoglobin. Note numerous target cells and spherocytes.
Figure 66. Peripheral blood film from patient with SC hemoglobinopathy showing target cells and poikilocytosis but no extreme sickled forms.

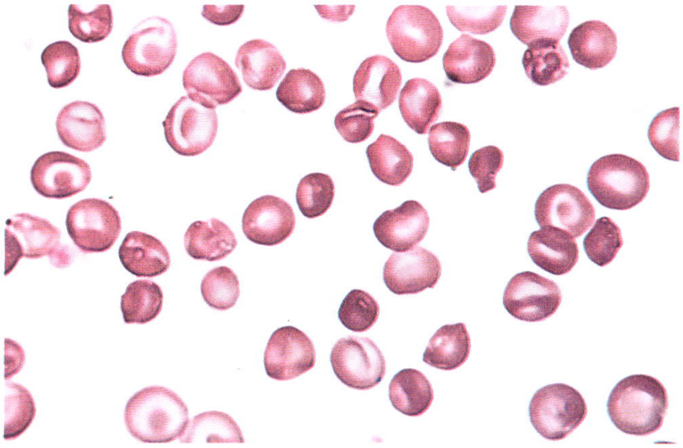

65

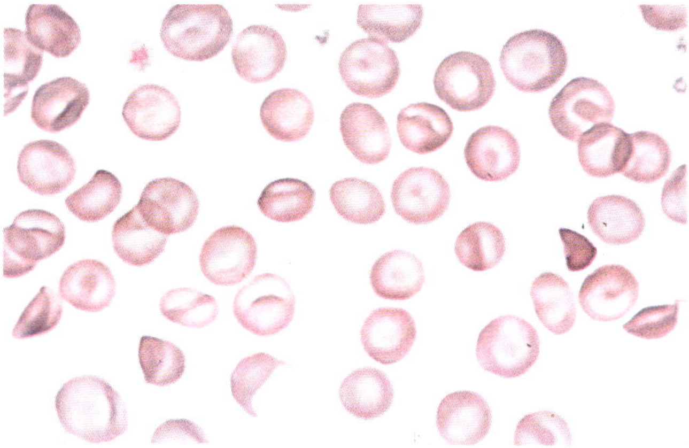

66

rubin from RBC breakdown may lead to cholelithiasis. On electrophoresis Hb S and C are seen in approximately equal amounts (Fig. 64).

Moderate or marked splenomegaly is found in approximately 66% of patients and may be more pronounced during crises. In contrast to those with sickle cell anemia, individuals with SC disease frequently have persistent splenomegaly throughout life. Although much less common than in sickle cell anemia, splenic infarcts may occur, especially during exposure to high altitudes, and some develop siderofibrotic nodules in the spleen.

Certain focal ischemic lesions, such as aseptic necrosis of the femoral head, retinal infarcts and renal papillary necrosis are seen with greater frequency in individuals with SC disease than in those with sickle cell anemia. While it has been postulated that the greater blood viscosity in SC disease accounts for the higher incidence of these focal lesions, it is likely that a patient's longevity is also a factor. These complications are most often seen at an age not attained by most patients with sickle cell anemia.

Bone Changes. Bone changes are similar to those seen in sickle cell anemia. Cortical thinning, coarsened trabeculation and evidence of bone infarction are common findings. Aseptic necrosis of the femoral head is seen more often than in sickle cell anemia, occurring in approximately 20% of adults with SC disease. Similar lesions of the humerus are also seen with greater frequency. In adolescents and adults the characteristic 'cod-fish vertebrae' may be seen. Salmonella osteomyelitis is a not infrequent complication in SC disease, as well as in sickle cell anemia.

Infection. While those with SC disease have a somewhat greater incidence of bacterial infections than seen in the population as a whole, the incidence is much less than in individuals with sickle cell anemia. The type of infection also differs somewhat between the two groups. While children with sickle cell anemia are prone to pyogenic bacterial infections often with overwhelming sepsis, in SC disease most are gram negative systemic infections, often with osteomyelitis. Pneumococcal sepsis and meningitis, common and life-threatening in sickle cell anemia, are rare in individuals with SC disease.

The Kidney. In SC disease, concentrating ability decreases with advancing age to reach ultimately, at about 50 years, the fixed maximum of 400-450 milliosmoles. While this pattern is also observed in individuals with AS hemoglobin, maximal concentrating capacity is more depressed in SC, for comparable age groups, and the fixed maximum is reached at a somewhat earlier age. This probably reflects the higher percentage of S hemoglobin and greater blood viscosity in SC as compared to AS subjects. Adults with Hb SC cannot acidify their urine below pH 5.3. This disturbance in acidifying capacity is greater than in AS subjects but less than in those with sickle cell anemia (see p. 51).

Microradioangiographic studies in adult SC kidneys reveal reduced numbers of vasa recta and loss of normal bundle architecture (Fig. 57B & C). These changes are similar to those observed in adults with AS hemoglobin.

Retinal Changes. Proliferative sickle retinopathy (PSR) is much more common in adults with SC disease (60-70%) than in those with sickle cell anemia (10%). Clinically symptomatic and significant stages of PSR are frequently observed in individuals with SC disease between 20 and 30 years of age. Peripheral arteriolar (and probably capillary) occlusion leads to neovascularization, the tuft of proliferating vessels resembling a "sea fan" (Fig. 62). Such neovascular abnormalities are most often seen in the superotemporal quadrant of the retina. Proliferative retinopathy is progressive and frequently leads to vitreous hemorrhages, retinal detachment and loss of vision.

"Black sunbursts" (black chorioretinal scars) which are commonly seen in adults with sickle cell anemia and probably result from small infarctions or hemorrhages, are seen in a smaller percentage of adults with SC disease (15-20%).

SC Disease and Pregnancy. Individuals with SC disease often become gravely ill during the third trimester. They may have frequent episodes of bone pain, and may develop pulmonary infarcts, congestive heart failure and hematuria. Severe anemia or shock may develop with dramatic suddenness, and some may die. While fertility does not appear to be impaired, fetal salvage is definitely decreased. This is the result of a high incidence of spontaneous abortions, stillbirths and neonatal deaths. There is also a high incidence of postpartum complications, including endometritis, pulmonary infarction, and fat embolism from marrow infarction. The normal fertility of patients with SC disease as well as the normal duration of their reproductive period result in a much higher incidence of pregnancies than in those with sickle cell anemia. This greater exposure to the stresses of pregnancy results in a greater number of complications.

Cardiovascular System. Heart size is normal and cardiac murmurs other than a soft systolic 'hemic' murmur are uncommon. Electrocardiograms are normal in uncomplicated SC disease.

The Liver. Although hepatocellular impairment is much more common in sickle cell anemia than in SC disease, hepatomegaly and abnormal liver function tests may also be seen in the latter. These findings may reflect serum hepatitis, fibrosis and/or hemosiderosis. Among older patients there is also an increased incidence of cholelithiasis.

Life Expectancy. No statistical data is available but individuals with SC disease have somewhat shortened survival times in comparison with normals. However, life expectancy is greater than in those with sickle cell anemia.

HEMOGLOBIN D

Hemoglobin D has the same electrophoretic mobility at pH 8.6 as Hb S, but does not sickle. It can be separated from S on agar gel electrophoresis at pH 6.0. The reported incidence of Hb D trait in American Blacks has varied from 0.085 to 0.4%; Hb D has also been described in Caucasians and East Indians.

Heterozygous individuals (AD) are completely asymptomatic and have no anemia. RBC morphology and RBC survival are normal.

The homozygous state (DD) is rare. There may be a mild degree of anemia with slight microcytosis and hypochromia. The most striking feature on examination of the peripheral blood smear is the large number of target cells (50-80%). RBC survival is slightly shortened but there is no significant disability associated with the homozygous state.

SD Hemoglobinopathy. This doubly heterozygous state is characterized by a relatively mild clinical course, some individuals being entirely asymptomatic. There may be arthralgia and/or abdominal pain, and splenic enlargement is noted in 1/3 of cases. Hemoglobin values of 8-10 gms % are usual, with some degree of reticulocytosis (approximately 10%). Characteristic features on peripheral smear include sickle forms, target cells, polychromasia and nucleated RBC. The diagnosis of SD hemoglobinopathy should be considered whenever the clinical course and degree of anemia are unusually mild for the homozygous S state. Although the sickle cell prep is positive and there is a single band of what appears to be S hemoglobin on electrophoresis at pH 8.6, the S and D components can be separated by agar gel electrophoresis at pH 6.0.

THE HIGH F GENE AND HEMOGLOBIN S

It is estimated that approximately 1/1,000 American and African Blacks possess the high F gene. This autosomal trait is characterized by increased amounts of hemoglobin F which persist throughout life. The F hemoglobin is distributed evenly in all RBC. These individuals are clinically normal and have no anemia. Heterozygotes have 15-35% F, the remainder being A hemoglobin, while the rare individuals who are homozygous for the high F gene have 100% F.

Those who are heterozygous for Hb S and also possess the high F gene have a very mild clinical course. Some are asymptomatic while others have occasional arthralgia only. Aseptic necrosis of the femoral head may occur but is uncommon. Hemoglobin F constitutes 15-35% of the total hemoglobin and S 65-85%, however, Hb F is uniformly distributed within the RBC. This is in contrast to sickle cell anemia where Hb F is heterogeneously distributed within the RBC (see Fig. 17). The presence of a significant amount of Hb F within each RBC impairs sickling, there being no sickling of these RBC at physiologic oxygen tensions. These doubly heterozygous individuals have a mild degree of hemolysis but are usually not anemic.

HEMOGLOBIN O ARAB

Hemoglobin O Arab is another less common β-chain variant, in which lysine is substituted for glutamic acid at the No. 121 position. Although this abnormal hemoglobin was first identified in an Arab family it is thought to have arisen in African peoples who previously inhabited what are now Arab territories. It has also been described in Jamaicans, Sudanese, Bulgarians and American Blacks. Electrophoretically Hb O Arab migrates as Hb C on paper but can be readily distinguished from C on agar gel at acid pH.

Heterozygous O Arab (AO). No clinical or hematologic abnormalities have been described in heterozygotes.

SO Disease. The interaction of Hb O Arab and Hb S enhances gelling. This doubly heterozygous state is characterized by a chronic hemolytic anemia and other clinical features indistinguishable from those of sickle cell anemia. The peripheral blood film characteristically shows extreme sickled forms as well as target cells, polychromasia and anisocytosis. This condition may be mistakenly diagnosed as SC disease if electrophoresis is done on filter paper rather than on agar gel at pH 6.2. However, the severe course of the disease and the presence of filamentous sickle forms on peripheral smear should lead one to suspect that SC is an incorrect diagnosis.

HEMOGLOBIN E

The distribution of the E gene is primarily throughout Southeast Asia. Hemoglobin E differs from A in the substitution of lysine for glutamine in the No. 26 position of the β-chain. The Hb E syndromes are generally mild unless in combination with thalassemia.

Heterozygous Hemoglobin E. The heterozygous state is completely asymptomatic. On examination of the peripheral blood smear an occasional target cell may be found.

Homozygous Hemoglobin E. First found in a Thai, hemoglobin E disease is very common throughout Southeast Asia. It is characterized by a mild to moderate hemolytic anemia and slight splenomegaly. Examination of the peripheral smear reveals numerous target cells (25-60%) as well as polychromasia. The diagnosis is established by hemoglobin electrophoresis which reveals only Hb E and a slight elevation of Hb F. Hb E moves similarly to Hb C and O Arab on paper and starch, but can be differentiated from them by agar gel electrophoresis at pH 6.1. (E migrates with A on the latter.)

SE Hemoglobinopathy. While Hb E and the thalassemias are widespread throughout Southeast Asia, other abnormal hemoglobins appear to be rare in this part of the world. Thus the combination of hemoglobins E and S is uncommon. This doubly heterozygous state was first described in the Eti-Turks, a small arabic-speaking group in southern Turkey who possess the highest incidence of Hb S (16.8%) in the white race. The incidence of Hb E in this group is reportedly 1-2%. A 70 year old Eti-Turk woman who had born 15 children was the first reported example of ES hemoglobinopathy. The latter is characterized by a mild hypochromic microcytic anemia. On electrophoresis there is approximately 40% Hb E and 60% Hb S.

Hemoglobin E—β-Thalassemia. Although the clinical picture is somewhat variable it is usually similar to that of β-thalassemia major. There is severe anemia, microcytosis and hypochromia, as well as many target cells, polychromasia, nucleated RBC, and basophilic stippling. Most have hepatosplenomegaly, growth and developmental retardation and an increased incidence of infections. Life span is reduced, many succumbing to parasitic or bacterial infections in childhood.

Hemoglobin electrophoresis reveals hemoglobins E and F, usually with no detectable A. A_2 cannot be quantitated in this condition, as hemoglobins E and A_2 have identical electrophoretic and chromatographic properties.

α-Thalassemia Associated With Hemoglobin E. Hemoglobin E and α-thalassemia are both very common in Southeast Asia and many different combinations of these disorders have been described. The hematologic findings and clinical symptoms vary considerably among the reported combinations, from a completely benign, asymptomatic state (eg.: α-thalassemia trait/Hb E trait) to a picture similar to that of β-thalassemia major (ex.: α-thalassemia$_1$/α-thalassemia$_2$/homozygous Hb E).

THE THALASSEMIA SYNDROMES AND S-THALASSEMIA

The Thalassemia syndromes are a group of genetically determined conditions affecting the synthesis of normal hemoglobin. They are mild in the heterozygote and severe in the homozygote. There is deficient synthesis of normal hemoglobin within the RBC, resulting from a defect in synthesis of either alpha

Figure 67. Peripheral blood film from child with S-thalassemia showing sickle forms, target cells and polychromasia. Note similarity to Fig. 41 (sickle cell anemia).

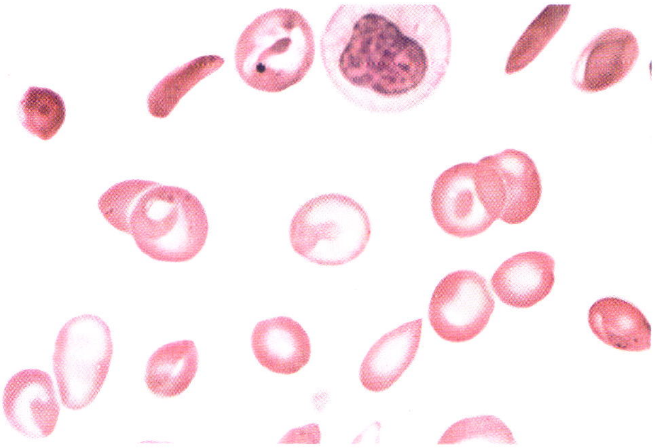

chains (α-thalassemia) or β-chains (β-thalassemia). This probably reflects a decrease or defect in messenger RNA directing chain synthesis.

β-thalassemia occurs with greatest frequency in the Po Valley, Sardinia, and other parts of the Mediterranean area. The α-thalassemia syndromes are most common in certain parts of Asia, but both are worldwide in distribution and affect most races. In American Blacks the incidence of β-thalassemia trait is estimated as 0.8% while the incidence of α-thalassemia trait has been reported as 1.55% in one U.S. city and 7.1% in another.

Thalassemia Major (Homozygous β-Thalassemia: Cooley's Anemia) is characterized by grossly defective synthesis of Hb A, impaired RBC production and increased hemolysis of the defective RBC. Affected individuals are dependent on repeated blood transfusions and most succumb before 20 years of age. Death is usually attributable to cardiac failure resulting from iron deposition in the myocardium.

β-Thalassemia Trait. Individuals with β-thalassemia trait (thalassemia minor) are asymptomatic. The condition is characterized by mild anemia and pallor. Some have slight splenomegaly. Hemoglobin values range from 9-13 gms %. Characteristic morphologic changes in RBC include hypochromia, microcytosis, aniso- and poikilocytosis, basophilic stippling and slight polychromasia. Mean corpuscular hemoglobin concentration (MCHC) is low ($<27\ \mu\mu g$). Ineffective erythropoiesis can be demonstrated by ferrokinetic studies with only 50-60% of the tracer iron injected appearing in the RBC mass within 14 days. Among individuals with β-thalassemia trait there is heterogeneity in relation to A_2 and fetal hemoglobin (either A_2 being elevated and hemoglobin F being normal, or the reverse), and also in relation to the degree of suppression of chain synthesis. In the doubly heterozygous state with the sickle gene, some produce no detectable hemoglobin A while others produce a subnormal amount.

Sickle β-Thalassemia (S-Thalassemia). Individuals with S-thalassemia have a moderately severe anemia and a clinical picture approaching that of sickle cell anemia. Vaso-occlusive episodes may be as frequent as in SS individuals; however, splenomegaly is often prominent and may persist throughout life. Examination of the peripheral blood smear reveals sickle cells, hypochromia and target cells (Fig. 67). On electrophoresis there may be 0-20% Hb A; those producing no Hb A have a more severe clinical picture. The percentage of fetal hemoglobin is variable, values of 1-26% being reported.

The α-Thalassemias. The α-thalassemias constitute several types of inherited defects in the production of α chains. The genetics are not completely understood, largely because of difficulties in defining the heterozygous states. However, these disorders seem to result from the interaction of at least 2 genes, a mild form designated α-thalassemia$_2$ and a more severe form, α-thalassemia$_1$. The production of α chains is suppressed, and as hemoglobins A, A_2 and F all contain α chains, there is no compensatory increase in A_2 and fetal hemoglobins. During fetal life the deficiency of α chains creates an excess of β and γ chains (see Chapter IV). These may form tetramers known as Bart's hemoglobin (γ^4) and hemoglobin H (β^4). Hemoglobin H is unstable and readily denatures within the RBC to form inclusion bodies.

The homozygous state (at least in the severe form) is incompatible with life as there is almost complete suppression of α chains, necessary components of all normal hemoglobins. Bart's hemoglobin, the predominant hemoglobin in homozygous α thalassemia, has a 10X greater affinity for oxygen than hemoglobin A and thus does not release oxygen at normal tissue O_2 tensions. Affected infants die *in utero* or at birth with a clinical picture resembling that of hydrops fetalis. This severe form has never been seen in Negroes, suggesting that this racial group has a *mild* thalassemia gene (or some other variation of genetic pattern).

The heterozygous state (*α-thalassemia trait*[s]) is the least severe of all the thalassemias. It is also the most difficult to detect after the first few months of life. These individuals are asymptomatic and hemoglobin values are normal or only slightly decreased (10-14 gms %). RBC morphology may be normal or there may be hypochromia, microcytosis and target cells, a picture resembling iron deficiency anemia. Osmotic fragility is decreased, serum iron is normal and there is no increase in A_2 or F hemoglobin. The diagnosis can be established at birth or in the first few months of life by demonstrating increased amounts of Bart's hemoglobin (5-20%) in the infants blood. However, as γ chain synthesis declines, Bart's hemoglobin disappears and α-thalassemia trait is extremely difficult to recognize with certainty in older children and adults. (This may be done by measuring rates of synthesis of α and β chains, but the techniques are too highly specialized for routine use at this time.)

Geographic Distribution

Agreement on the incidence and geographical distribution of the sickle cell gene is dependent on the reliability of diagnostic tests for the specific identification of Hb S (see page 72). The World Health Organization Technical Report Series has been updating frequency data since 1966.

The fundamental genetic aberrations of all hemoglobinopathies exhibiting genetic transmission are due to mutations, deletions, or crossing over. Mutations are the result of the substitution of amino acids in the hemoglobin molecule by other amino acids. Hemoglobin S is a classical example of this type since the only difference from Hb A is the substitution of valine for glutamic acid in the 6th position from the N-terminal end of the beta chain. Deletion is the result of a missing fragment of DNA typified by Hb Gun Hill where the 91st through the 95th amino acids are missing. Leiden and Freiburg hemoglobins lack one amino acid. Crossing over may be exemplified by Hb Lepore where much of the molecule is identical to the nonalpha chain of Hb A_2 while the other part is homologous to the beta chain. The assumption is that there must have been an unequal crossing over between delta and beta genes and would imply an area of contiguity of these genes on the chromosome. A detailed discussion of abnormal hemoglobin structures and their relation to genetically transmitted clinical states can be found in an article by Beuzard, et al.

HEMOGLOBIN S

Hemoglobin S in the homozygous and heterozygous states is of primary concern and is rather widely distributed (Fig. 68). Sickling from this hemoglobin is more devastating than any other abnormal hemoglobin form. Assuming that approximately 10% of Negroes in the United States have the sickle cell trait, Neel has calculated the frequency of sickle cell anemia (homozygous) at birth to be 2.8 per 1,000 births. A carrier incidence of 8 to 10% of Negroes studied in the United States is reported with up to

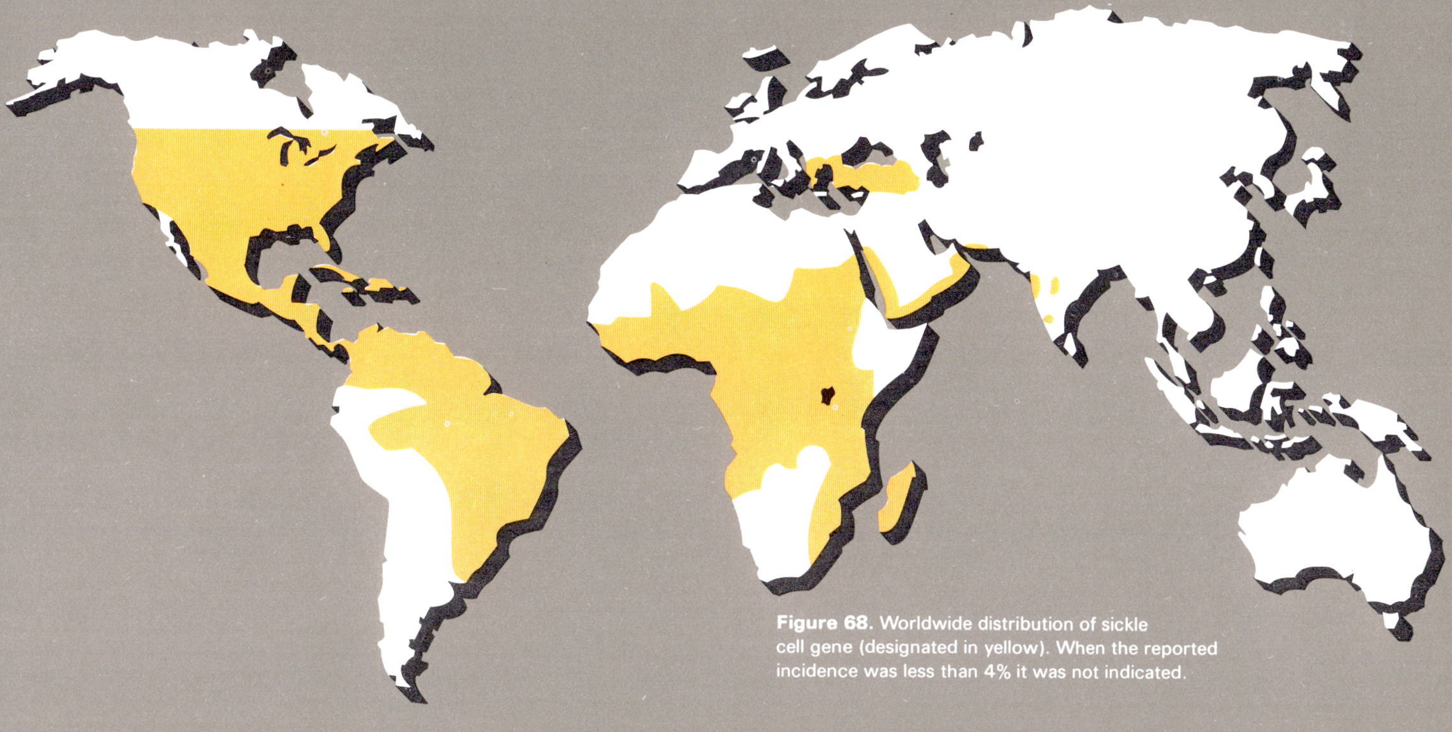

Figure 68. Worldwide distribution of sickle cell gene (designated in yellow). When the reported incidence was less than 4% it was not indicated.

14% among 1,000 adults tested in South Carolina. The incidence at birth must have been higher. Incidence among African Negroes exists within considerable ranges (Fig. 69). Frequency is highest in a belt extending from west to east across the middle third of Africa. The average frequency of the sickling trait appears to be around 20%. In addition, there is considerable variation among African tribes. In Uganda ranges from 2.9% to 46% frequency is reported from studies of different ethnological groups. However, the West Coast can be considered more comparable in climate to the United States and the incidence appears to be from 12.4% in the Gold Coast to 27% in Sierra Leone (Fig. 69).

Sickling and the incidence of Hb S is by no means uncommon in Northern Mediterranean Countries (Fig. 69 and 70). Not all of the sickling reported is due to Hb S. The reported sickle cell trait incidence in the Lake Copais area of Greece appears unexplainable on the basis of Negro admixture alone. In addition, the blood groups of these people do not differ significantly from other people of Greece but the cDe or R_0 chromosome is less common than among African Negroes. Arabian and certain groups of South Indian people also have Hb S (Fig. 68 and 69).

Increasing reports on the distribution of the sickle cell gene, such as those from Central and South America (Fig. 68) have made explanation of genetic transmission by way of long term racial origins difficult. However, modern interpretation of inheritance still favors that first advanced by Neel.

The incidence of the hemoglobin S gene among individuals in certain areas in Africa is two to three times the incidence found in the United States. Either genetic differences of a morbid nature, separate but linked to sickle cell anemia, or other lethal conditions, endemic to areas where sickle cell anemia occurs, must be invoked to explain the apparent separation of the Black race into these two groups. Something must account for the maintenance of the high incidence of the sickle cell gene in African populations. The manifestation of the sickling crisis may be expected in 1 of 50 homozygous S people in the United States, whereas the clinical picture appears in less than 1 in 1,000 in Africa. Perhaps better diagnostic procedures and clinical reports will dispel some of these differences. However, the relation of malarial incidence and glucose-6-phosphate dehydrogenase deficiency gene frequencies in endemic areas of Africa cannot be overlooked.

MALARIAL RESISTANCE

Considerable genetic resistance to malaria in man apparently can be conferred by major genes for abnormal hemoglobins and by other conditions. It has been well established that the sickle cell gene does protect against malarial infestation. Articles by Allison are most illuminating in this regard. In addition, Allison described the likely relationship of glucose-6-phosphate dehydrogenase (G6PD) deficiency gene to resistance against malaria. The distribution of the sickle cell gene and the G6PD deficiency gene can be largely superimposed on the areas of high malarial occurence (Figs. 69 and 70). Accumulation of the sickle cell gene in high incidence levels cannot be accounted for by genetic mutation. Natural selection should tend to eliminate or hold down the gene incidence because death by sickle cell anemia (homozygous) removes two genes from the pool. Malaria, however, also causes a great deal of illness and mortality among infants within areas where the sickle cell gene is prevalent. Newborns have low malarial parasite counts because they are less exposed to mosquitos, acquire some transplacental immunity, and have higher levels of fetal hemoglobin as a protection against parasite growth, among many other causes.

Figure 69. Distribution of selected hemoglobinopathies in Africa and Asia. Note areas of overlapping incidence and compare with Fig. 70.

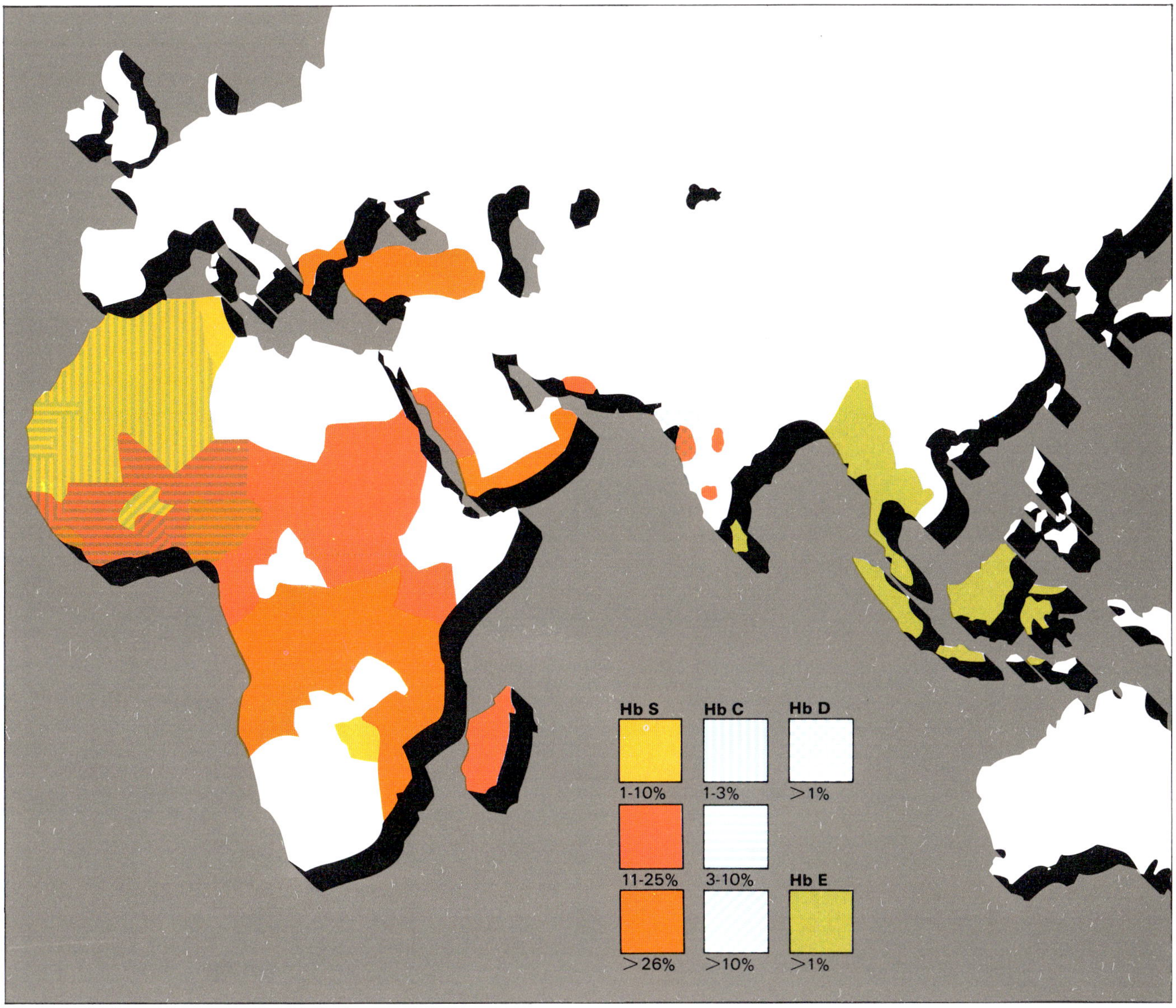

Mortality due to malaria is not significant in older children and adults because of acquisition of self-immunity. However it should be noted that malarial infection can be very severe in some patients. The majority of deaths occur within the first two years of life.

Sickle cell trait children show infestation by malarial parasites at the same rate as non sickle cell trait children. However, presence of the abnormal

Figure 70. Distribution of Falciparum malaria and G6PD deficiency in Africa and Asia. Compare with Fig. 69 and note areas of overlapping incidence.

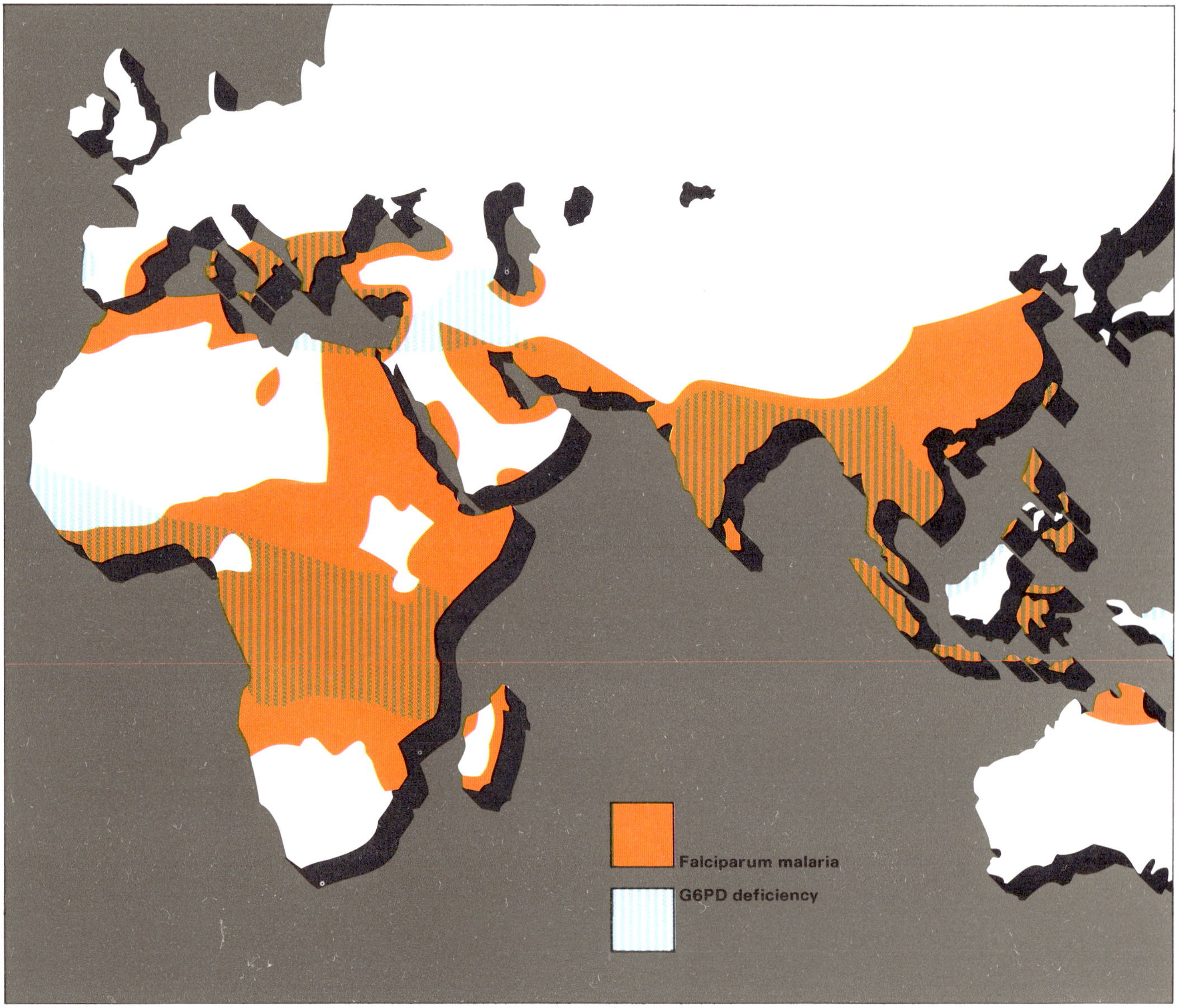

sickle cell hemoglobin limits multiplication of trophozoites so that parasite counts remain low. Immunity against malaria develops dramatically during one to four years of life and among children of this age fewer sickle cell carriers show parasites. Parasite counts are also found to be significantly lower. Mortality from malaria is higher in subjects without sickle cell trait. In addition, parasite counts are lower in subjects having high concentration of Hb S (homozygotes), at intermediate levels in heterozygotes, and highest in normal subjects where no Hb S occurs.

The mechanism of protection against malaria afforded by sickle cell hemoglobin is not well understood. Suggestions include sickling and phagocytic removal of red cells containing parasites, and that *P. falciparum* may be unable to effectively utilize sickle cell hemoglobin. These suggestions may also account for protection against malaria by other abnormal hemoglobins, such as thalassemia, and other abnormalities such as G6PD deficiency. Metabolic pathways are slowed when the G6PD enzyme is deficient. It is unlikely that malarial parasites can attain maximal growth in enzyme deficient cells. The deficiency is inherited as a sex-linked gene with full expression in hemizygous males and homozygous females and with partial expression in heterozygous females. About 11% of United States Negro males carry this red cell abnormality. Frequencies above 2% in Old World areas are shown in Figure 70. The presence of this abnormality in conjunction with sickle cell hemoglobin provides considerable protection against malaria and can account for the persistence and increased frequency of the sickle cell gene in Old World populations. Sickle cell heterozygotes and homozygotes occur in expected random mating frequency in infants but there is a significant increase in heterozygotes at reproduction age. Sickle cell gene carriers enjoy a favorable position to survive to reproductive age. This event, however, does not alleviate the devasting effects of sickle cell anemia in the homozygote or when heterozygous with Hb C.

Abortions and premature births occur more frequently with malarial infection than with sickle cell trait. This affords an apparent increased fertility rate among sickle cell carriers (see p. 56). Coupled with protection against malarial death due to interference with parasite growth and increased gamma globulin levels for immunity against malaria, the apparent increased fertility allows increased sickle cell gene frequency. This condition continues until the advantage afforded by the heterozygote is counterbalanced by the disadvantage of the homozygote. A new stable equilibrium is then maintained. The high gene frequencies are only attained where malaria is hyperendemic or holoendemic.

Resistance against malaria by the sickle cell trait is an example of a large number of mutations affecting protein structure that will provide unfavorable conditions for particular disease states. Mutant genes would increase in frequency due to their selective advantage. This form of resistance seems to be widespread in the biological world.

HEMOGLOBIN C

The presence of Hb C genes, such as occurs in West Africa, would likely be mutually exclusive with sickle cell genes (Fig. 69). When Hb C gene rises, the incidence of sickle cell genes falls (see Ghana and Upper Volta in West Africa). Both of these genes are known to be disadvantageous in combination with thalassemia. Neither gene can reach high frequencies in populations where thalassemia is common (a broad belt including Mediterranean shores, Persian Gulf, Arabian Sea and South China Sea).

HEMOGLOBIN E

In Asia Hb E is common. The highest frequencies (15-30%) exist in Burma, Cambodia, Ceylon, Indonesia and Malaysia (Fig. 69).

While the incidence of Hb E among the Eti-Turks is only 1-2%, the incidence of Hb S is 16.8% in this group. Thus most instances of SE hemoglobinopathy have been reported in Eti-Turks.

Hemoglobin Detection and Identification

Detection and quantitation of hemoglobin has been standard laboratory practice since the first decade of the 20th century, although methods and reference bases have been disputed and modified for greatest clinical value.

Within the last 25 years, recognition that distinct hemoglobin variations were the basis of hereditary anemias demanded development of techniques to identify these specific hemoglobin types. One investigator, Stamatoyannopoulas, lists over 40 abnormal hemoglobins known to be due to changes in the alpha chain and more than 80 due to changes in the beta chain.

SICKLING AT THE MOLECULAR LEVEL

The molecular era for the study of sickle cell disease emanates from experimental observations beginning with the identification of Hb S as a molecular anomaly by Pauling and co-workers in 1949. Serious students of hemoglobin molecular abnormalities should refer to the work of Harris, Hunt, Ingram, Konigsberg, Braunitzer, and Perutz. The precise molecular data provided by these investigators led directly to the development of a molecular hypothesis for sickling of erythrocytes containing Hb S by Murayama in 1964. He constructed a precision three dimensional scale model of the hemoglobin molecule and drew inferences from the molecular data available (Fig. 1). He modified his hypothesis to arrive at precise specific descriptions of the molecular events taking place during the stacking of Hb S tetramers and the deformation of erythrocytes containing this abnormal form of hemoglobin. Practical use of such information has been developed by Nalbandian and co-workers for diagnosis and treatment of sickle cell disease. Our intent is to describe the molecular background details leading to specific diagnostic procedures and provide protocols for the tube tests and automated tests useful for individual diagnosis or mass screening programs.

Murayama described the hemoglobin molecule as a truncated tetrahedron composed of two alpha chains and two beta chains. The chains have a mirrored symmetry with reference to a central molecular axis. When deoxygenation occurs the beta chains displace laterally about 7 Angstrom units (Fig. 71). Upon oxygenation again the beta chains shift back toward the central axis of symmetry (Fig. 72). Hemoglobin S differs from Hb A by an amino acid substitution of valine for glutamic acid in the sixth position from the amino end of each beta chain. Murayama hypothesized that the valine in its surface position becomes available for the formation of hydrophobic interactions with some yet unidentified position on the alpha chains of other hemoglobin tetramers (Fig. 73). However, for stacking of molecules to result, the tetramers must be in a deoxygenated form so that a steric fit can be accomplished (Fig. 74). Oxygenation would once again eliminate the steric fit and stacking would be reversed or prevented. Murayama and Hasegawa further proposed that a low molecular weight nonprotein cofactor interacts between stacking tetramers since the hydrophobic bonding can be prevented by dialysis (Fig. 75). Stacking of hemoglobin S molecules will continue in the deoxygenated state until long helical monofilaments are formed (Fig. 76). Six membered microcables will then form by lateral aggregation (Fig. 77). Eventually all of the hemoglobin in the RBC will be in the form of these superhelices filling the spaces made available by the dynamic motion of the cell membrane. These processes lead to the distorted or "sickled" cell (Figs. 2, 4 and 5). Fetal hemoglobin, methemoglobin, and perhaps other atypical hemoglobin molecules may

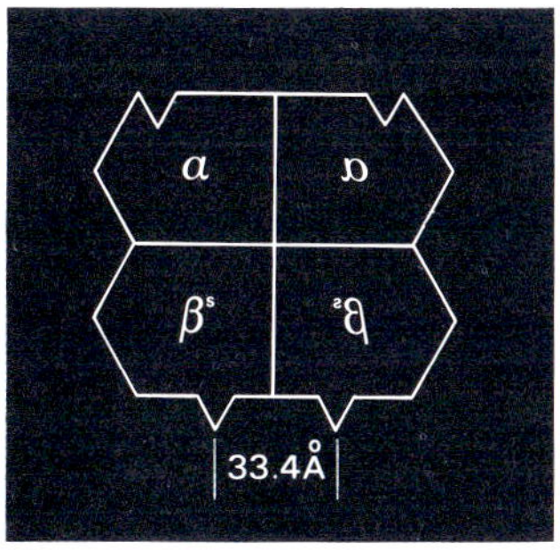

71

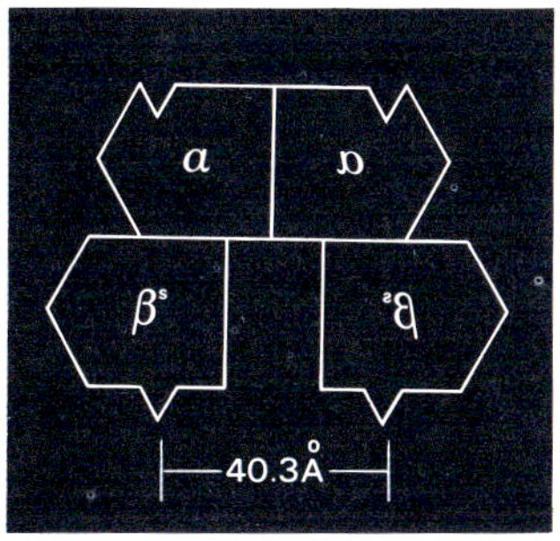

72

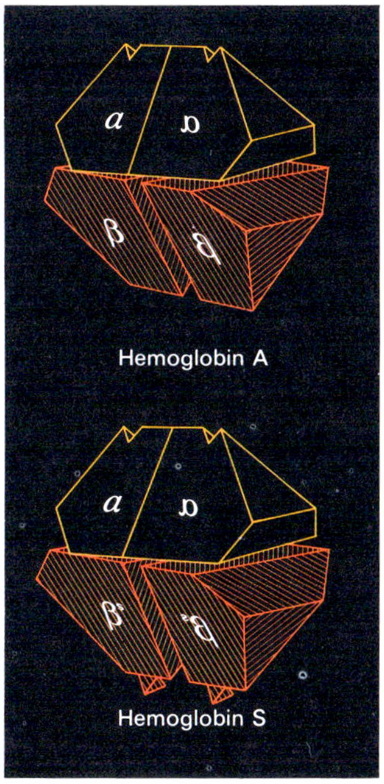

73

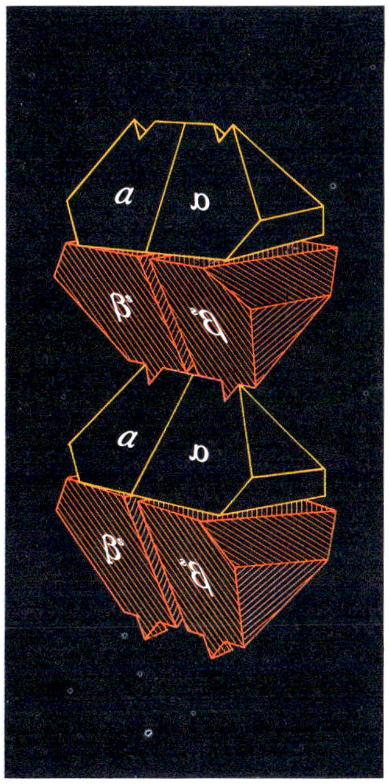

74

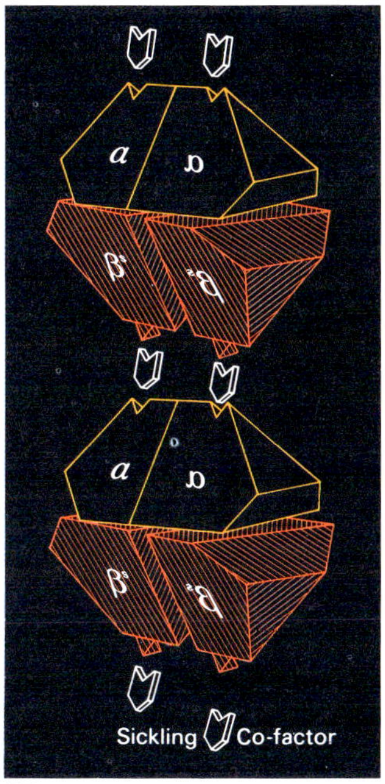

75

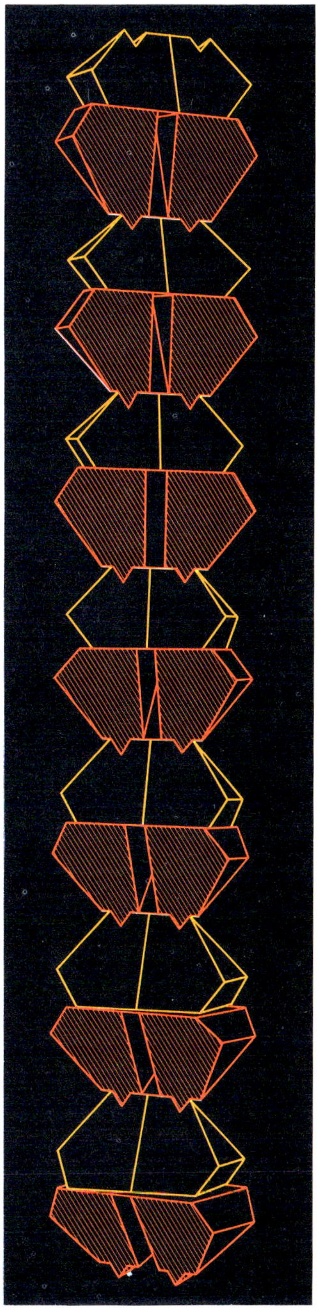

76

Figure 71. Schematic representing configuration of Hb S in the oxygenated state. Comparison with Fig. 72 indicates a medial shift of the β chains. Movement may be hinge-like rather than parallel displacement as shown in these diagrams.

Figure 72. Schematic representing configuration of Hb S induced by deoxygenation. Beta chains are displaced laterally as compared to the oxygenated state depicted in Fig. 71.

Figure 73. Truncated tetrahedron representations of hemoglobins A and S derived from a precision scale model by Dr. Makio Murayama, National Institutes of Health, Bethesda, Maryland. Protrusions shown at the base of the β chains represent valine substituted for glutamic acid in the 6th position from the N-terminal end.

Figure 74. Interacting tetramers of deoxygenated Hb S molecules. Note that the β chains are shown displaced laterally and that the tabs representing valine on the β chains sterically fit complimentary notches on α chains of a second molecule.

Figure 75. Tetramer-tetramer linkage Hb S mediated by a dialyzable cofactor capable of inducing hydrophobic interactions between the deoxygenated molecules.

Figure 76. Interacting Hb S tetramers to form a long chain microfilament. Dialyzable sickling cofactors are not shown at the hydrophobic sites of interaction.

Figure 77. Microfilaments aggregated laterally to form a microcable. Note the usual six microfilaments in the microcable.

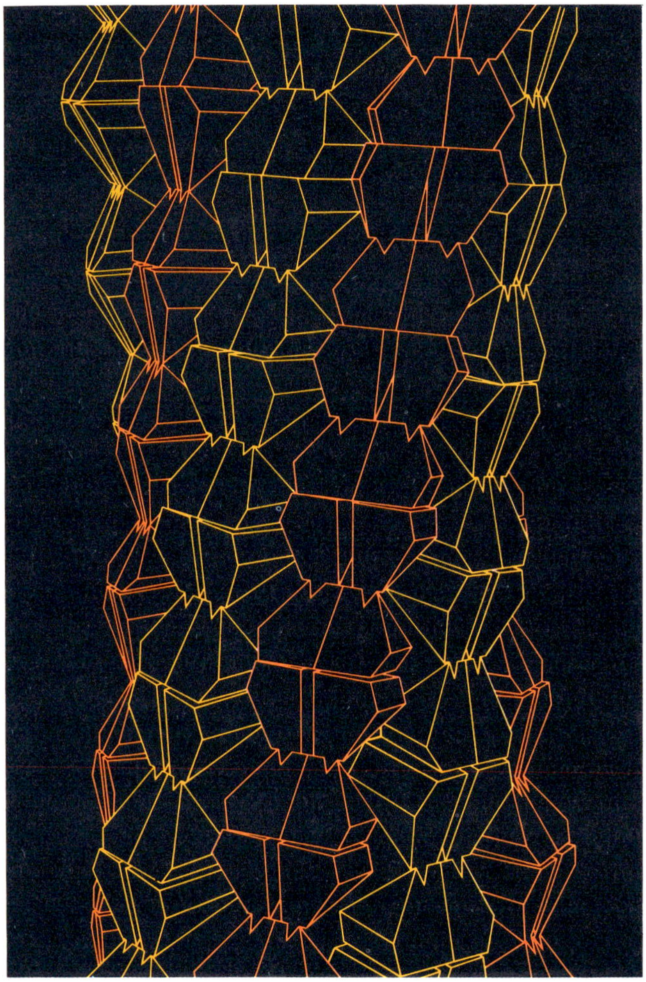

be present in the cell matrix but do not participate in the tetramer-tetramer hydrophobic interactions. Sufficient quantities of such molecules may prevent the physical cell shape change even though some molecular hemoglobin aggregations occur intracellularly upon deoxygenation. Inferences by deduction from molecular precision of the Murayama hypothesis has provided newly developed specific tests for Hb S.

Figure 78. Stability of proteins in aqueous media. Thermal inversion curve of hemoglobin constructed from data published by Scheraga and colleagues. Hemoglobin S has a temperature maximum of stability near 37° C. Hydrophobic bonds are decreased in strength while hydrogen bond strength increases as the temperature approaches zero.

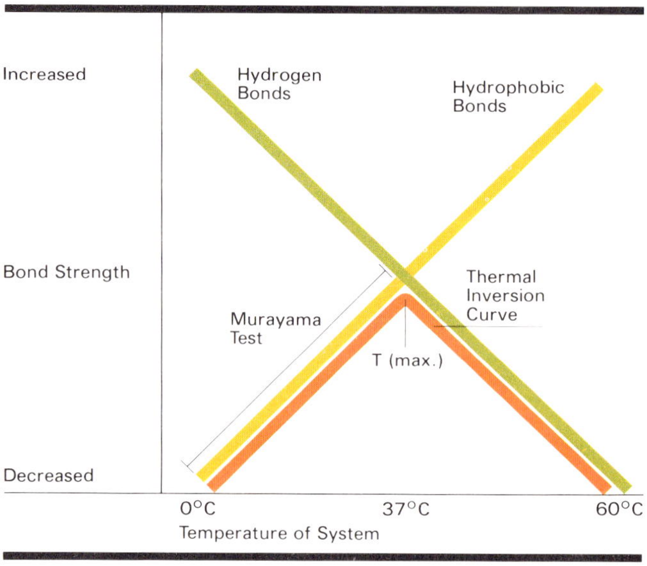

The Murayama Test. The strength of hydrogen bonds and hydrophobic interactions of proteins in aqueous systems behave in a reciprocal manner as derived from the data of Scheraga (Fig. 78). Hydrophobic interactions decrease in strength as the temperature falls while hydrogen bond strength increases. When the temperature rises above the optimum for any given protein, hydrogen bonds are weakened and primary protein structure is lost. Hydrophobic interactions therefore lose stability as well. If Murayama's hypothesis is correct, deoxygenated hemoglobin S hemolysates at 37° C and should be in a gel state due to the hemoglobin tetramer interactions. This was found to be the case (Fig. 79). When such gels are brought to 0° C they should liquefy even when maintained in the deoxygenated condition. This also was found to be the case (Fig. 80). Return toward 37° C brought about gelation once again. In effect, these experiments were designed to encompass events on the left arm of the thermal inversion curve for hemoglobin S (Fig. 78). Gel formation

Figure 79. Hemolysate of deoxygenated Hb S at 37° C; positive Murayama Test. Molecular hemoglobin interactions to form the gel are reversible when the temperature approaches 0° C but will reform again when brought back to 37° C.

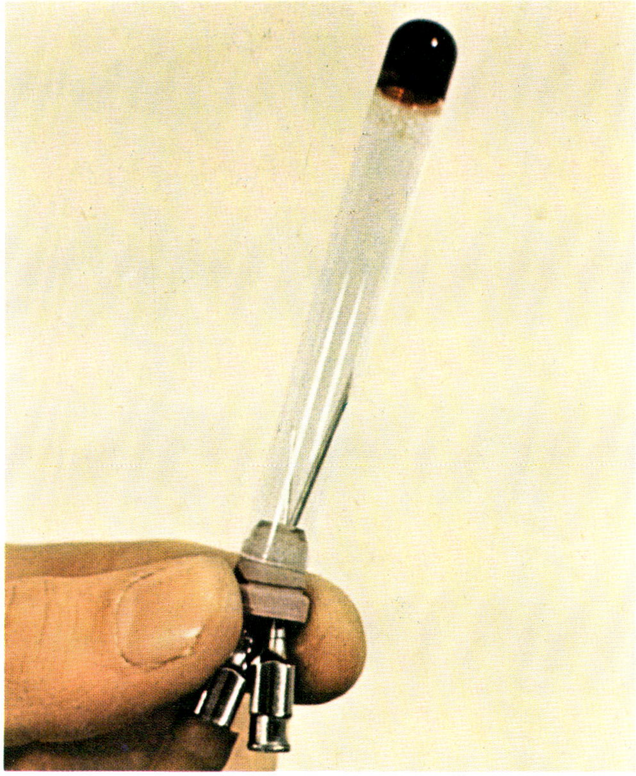

was due to hydrophobic interactions since bonding was lost when the hemolysate was brought to 0° C, while hydrogen bonds gained in strength. Nalbandian designed a specific test for hemoglobin S on the basis of this information and named it "The Murayama Test." The test is performed on stromata-free, concentrated, deoxygenated hemolysates. Predictions were made, and later confirmed, that hemoglobin C (Harlem), a structural variant of hemoglobin S, would give a positive Murayama Test, while other sickling hemoglobins such as C (Georgetown) and Hb I would be negative.

The Murayama Test is not suitable for mass screening procedures, but is useful as a research tool. Agents suspected to prevent or reverse hemoglobin S aggregation under conditions of the test can be added at 0 ° C. If effective, gelation will not occur when the hemolysate is brought to room temperature. Urea was found to be such an agent. These observations led to the proposal that urea would be an effective chemotherapeutic agent. In addition, these observations led to diagnostic tube tests and automated procedures, specific for Hb S and the rare structural variant C (Harlem), useful for individual or screening studies.

AVAILABLE TESTS AND RELIABILITY

Low solubility tests, electrophoresis, amino acid sequencing, and genetic data have led to the identification of at least 160 hemoglobin variants. The very existence of multiple variants, and the likelihood of many more to be uncovered, has demanded the development of rapid specific diagnostic tests. Most tests proposed are nonspecific and unreliable when used alone. A combination of tests has been necessary for the specific identification of a given hemoglobinopathy. Even so, false negative results in the initial test will miss important hemoglobin variants.

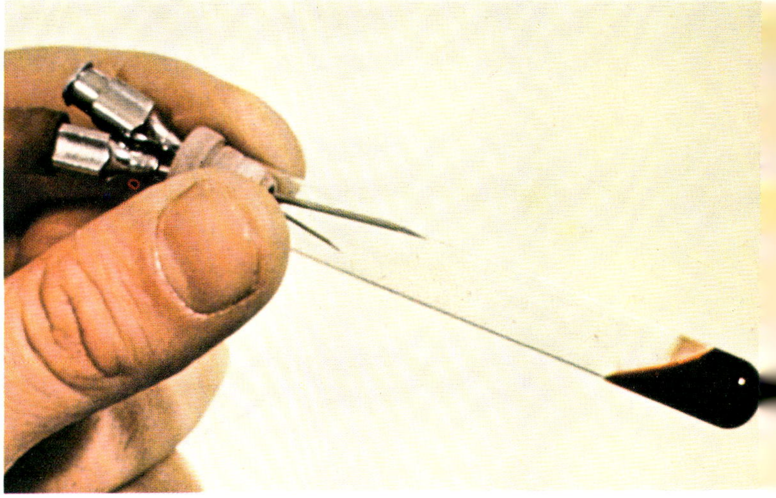

Figure 80. Hemolysate of deoxygenated Hb S at 0° C. The gel formed at 37° C is reversed at 0° C by reduction of hydrophobic bond strength. See also Fig. 78 and 79.

Human hemoglobinopathies S and C (Harlem) have a common mechanism for sickling. However, other hemoglobinopathies differ in their manner of sickling and none are similar to animal types. There is no logical animal model for the study of sickling. (Reproduced or modified by permission from Makio Murayama.

Table B
Hemoglobinopathies manifesting sickled erythrocytes

Human origin	Nonhuman origin
S	Deer
C (Harlem)	Sheep
C (Georgetown)	Goat
I	Mongoose
Bart's	Raccoon
Alexandra	Hamster
Memphis/S	Squirrel
Pôrto Alegre	

False positive initial results are at first alarming but further identification will clarify results. Consequences of the unreliability of diagnostic tests for abnormal hemoglobins are undiagnosed cases, undue alarm and unnecessary treatment, erroneous diagnosis of sickle cell anemia for some other less hazardous condition, and the burden of incorrect statistics.

Available diagnostic tests for hemoglobinopathy include erythrocyte sickling tests, low solubility tests, electrophoresis, and hemoglobin determination. Further specific identification is afforded by sequential amino acid analysis and other sophisticated methods of protein characterization. Common reasons for the unreliability of these tests include: 1) collection of blood samples within four months after transfusion, 2) incorrect labeling of specimens, 3) lack of quality control in methods, 4) long sample storage, exposure to heat, bacterial contamination, and drying during testing, 5) exceeding 2% sodium metabisulfite and not using the reagent freshly prepared, and 6) confusion of poikilocytosis for sickling. In addition, sampling of blood too early in the neonatal period before sufficient B chains are involved in the synthesis of hemoglobin renders sickling preparations and solubility tests unreliable.

SICKLING PREPARATIONS

Based on the observation that reduced oxygen tension promotes sickling of Hb S or AS erythrocytes the "sickle prep" has been used as a screening test for many years. A drop of blood is placed on a glass slide and mixed with a drop of fresh 2% sodium metabisulfite (reducing agent). The preparation is cover slipped and rimmed with petroleum jelly to prevent drying. Sickled forms are usually noted within 15 minutes if Hb S is present. While sickling will be observed in both homozygous S and AS samples, the shape of the sickled cells differs somewhat. The homozygous state produces a characteristic long pointed sickle cell while the heterozygous state does not (Fig. 81 Aand B). In the latter only holly-leaf forms are characteristically observed.

The physico-chemical reasons for sickling may vary for different abnormal sickling hemoglobins. For example, Hb S, by far the most common sickling hemoglobin, or Hb C (Harlem) likely involve hydrophobic interactions while others, such as Hb C (Georgetown) likely involve covalent bonding. Listed in Table B are several abnormal human hemoglobins and a number of animal hemoglobins that manifest sickling *ex vivo*. (None of the animal hemoglobins resemble Hb S in their molecular basis for sickling, and thus, animal models for the study of sickle cell anemia do not exist.)

SOLUBILITY TESTS

Tube Tests. A series of modifications of low solubility tests, first introduced by Itano in 1953, led to the development of a urea-dithionite tube test for the specific identification of Hb S. A dithionite tube test is first performed with the reagents, sodium dithionite, potassium phosphate, and saponin. RBC lyse, when introduced into the reagent mixture, the released hemoglobin is deoxygenated, and the beta chains of each molecule are displaced laterally. When

Figure 81. Sickling preparations viewed by ordinary light microscopy. **A.** Filamentous sickle forms developed in Hb SS blood. **B.** Holly leaf forms developed in Hb AS blood. (unstained, X 1800).

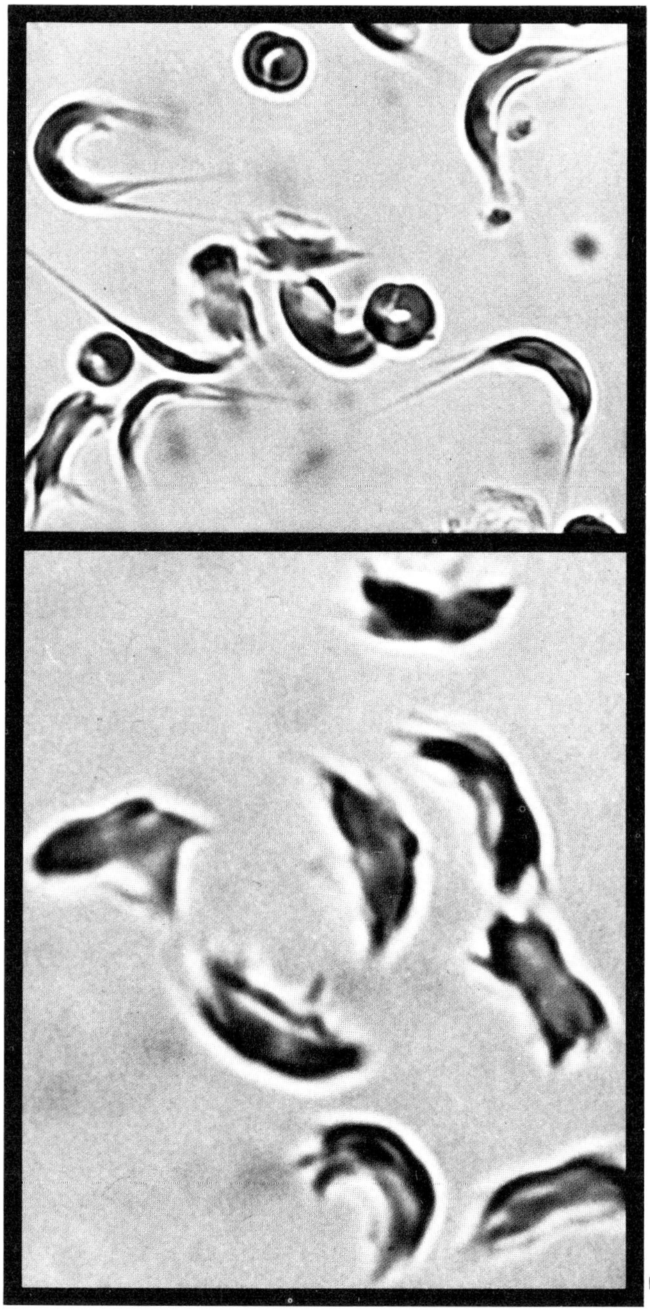

A

B

Hb S or C (Harlem) is present, molecular stacking will occur due to hydrophobic interactions. A nematic liquid crystal system of microfilaments and microcables will impart turbidity to the system with light scattering properties so that objects cannot be visualized through the system. Other sickling hemoglobins (for example, Hb C [Georgetown] Hb I, Hb Bart's) will form turbidity due to low solubility in the system but for reasons other than hydrophobic interactions. In either case, the test is positive (Fig. 82). Negative tests, such as for Hb A, do not develop turbidity and light scattering (Fig. 82). The test, completed in 5 minutes, only requires 20 gamma of blood which can be taken from a finger or ear prick sample.

Specific identification of Hb S can be made by adding urea to the positive dithionite test result. If the turbidity is due to hydrophobic interactions, as will be the case with Hb S, the test result will revert to negative in the presence of urea (Fig. 83). If the turbidity is due to other bonding, such as electrostatic, in the case of rare sickling hemoglobins other than Hb S, the positive test result will persist in the presence of urea (Fig. 84). The tube tests are rapid and inexpensive but still require manual manipulations. They are suitable for individual testing or testing where automated equipment is not available.

Solubility tests, with or without the urea modification, cannot distinguish SS hemoglobin from the trait, AS, or from any other hemoglobin combination with Hb S, such as SC, SD, etc. In addition, other hemoglobin types such as C or D without combination with S will not be detected. Whenever Hb S is identified by a solubility test, electrophoresis and other suitable identification procedures should be used in follow-up work.

Automated Tests. Identical molecular considerations utilized in the tube tests have been applied to automated systems. Anticoagulated whole blood

Figure 82. Positive and negative dithionite tube tests. The negative test (on the left) shows no interference with light transmission. Hemoglobins with low solubility in the test reagents will have interference with light transmission and the test is considered positive (on the right). Hemoglobin S forms a nematic liquid crystal system in the deoxygenated conditions of the test.

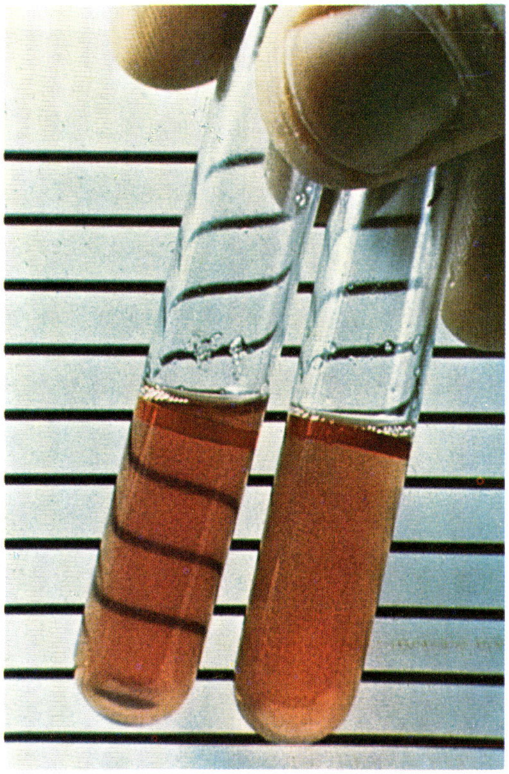

Figure 83. Two stage procedure of the urea-dithionite test. Hemoglobin S gives a positive dithionite tube test (**A**) but becomes negative when introduced into identical reagents with urea added (**B**). Urea disperses the nematic liquid crystal system formed by hydrophobic interactions.

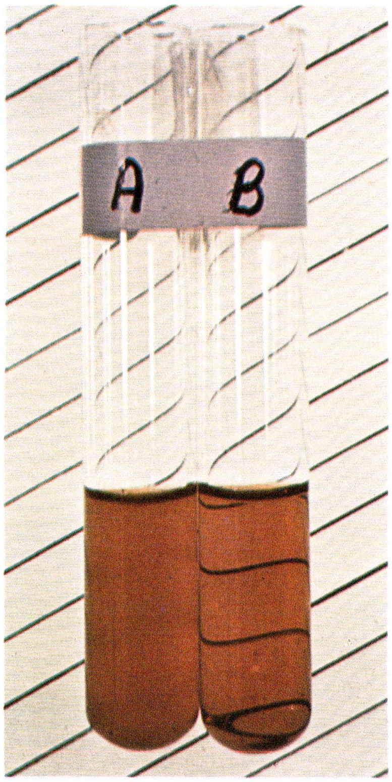

Figure 84. A positive dithionite tube test (**A**) produced by a non-S sickling hemoglobin. When introduced into identical reagents with urea added (**B**) the test remains positive. Low solubilities from non-S sickling hemoglobins are not formed by hydrophobic interactions so that urea has no effect on the interference of light transmittance.

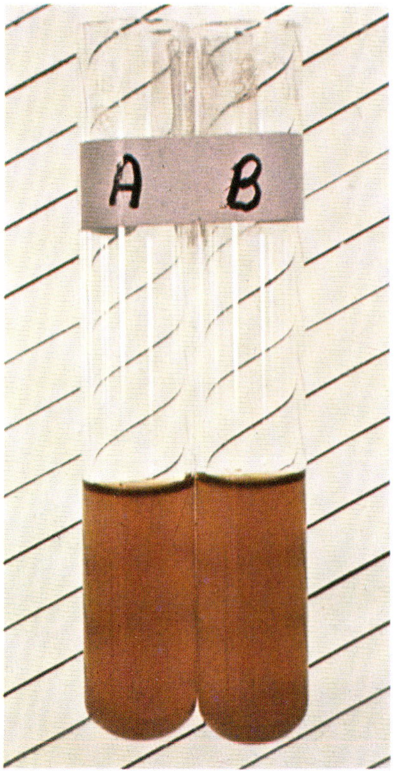

samples are introduced into sequential multiple autoanalyzer systems. Reagents induce deoxygenation and the formation of nematic liquid crystal systems as in the tube test, except that transmittance of light through the test system is measured objectively by a colorimeter and recorded electronically. Low solubility hemoglobins interfere with light transmittance to a greater extent than hemoglobins such as Hb A that are soluble in the test reagents (Fig. 85). If a second parallel line with added urea is run, the nematic liquid crystal system will disperse due to the interference with hydrophobic interactions by urea. A normal transmittance of light will then occur (Fig. 86); in other words, a positive test result will be converted to a normal pattern. This conversion will only occur when Hb S or its structural variant, Hb C (Harlem), is present. When some other rare non-S sickling variant is present, it will be detected in the line without urea and interference with light transmission will not be reversed in the line with urea.

The automated test just described will specifically identify Hb S or C (Harlem) as well as a collective identification of non-S sickling hemoglobins at the rate of 480 whole blood specimens per technician per day. An accelerated automated dithionite test has been developed to handle 1,200 specimens per technician per day at a reagent cost of about 0.2¢ each. Electronic amplification enhances the diagnostic differences in curves from positive and negative specimens (Fig. 87). Electrophoresis should be used to further identify the hemoglobin types uncovered by positive automated results.

Automated solubility tests have the same precautions and limitations noted for the tube solubility tests.

HEMOGLOBIN ELECTROPHORESIS

Hemoglobin electrophoresis is a useful tool for identification of specific hemoglobin types. As established by Tiselius, proteins can be separated and classified according to their surface charge and migration in an electric field. When hemoglobin (or other protein) molecules are in solution, partial ionization takes place and a net electrical charge is acquired. The latter depends not only on the number of uncombined ionizable groups in the molecule but also on the pH of the solution. Amino acid substitutions in the various abnormal hemoglobins result in various net charges in solution. These differences can be used to separate the abnormal hemoglobins on the basis of their movement in an electrical field. The RBC hemolysate is placed at a starting point and an electric current is applied across the field of

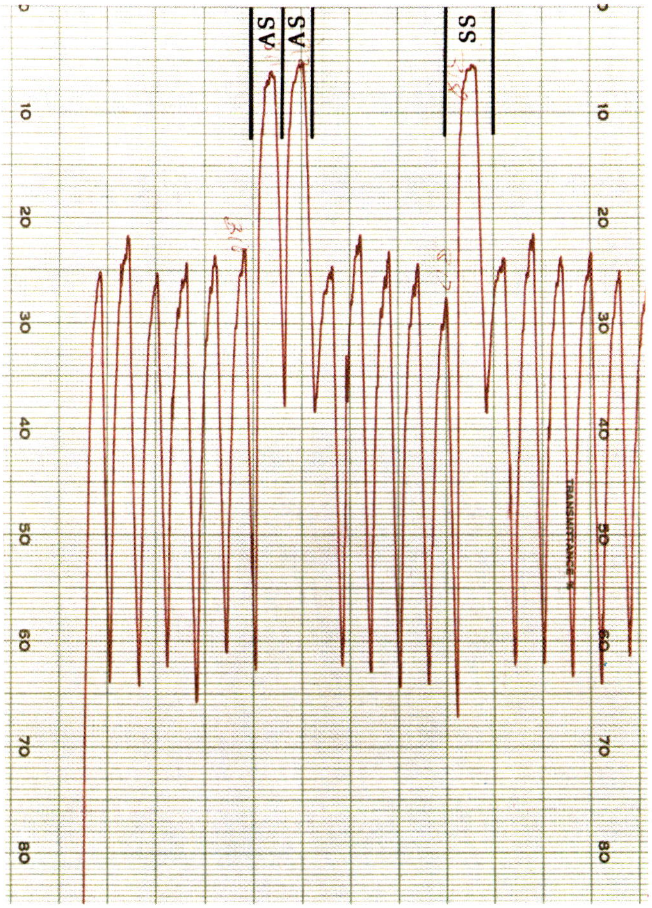

Figure 85. Typical curve by the automated dithionite test. The presence of Hb S in either homozygous or heterozygous states reduces light transmittance as compared to samples containing no Hb S.

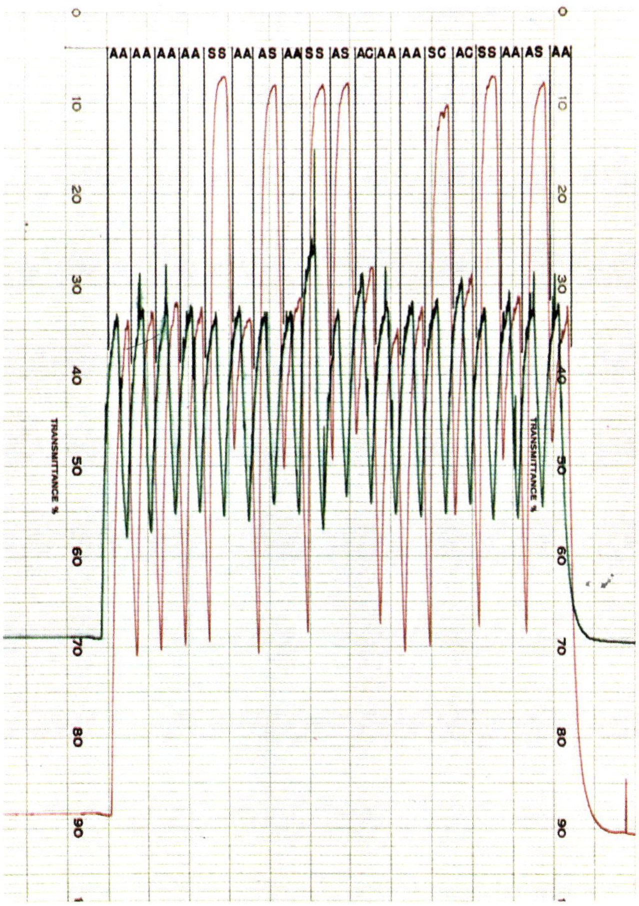

Figure 86. Typical curve by the automated urea-dithionite test. Whenever Hb S is present light transmission is reduced (red tracing). The same hemoglobin in the line with urea and dithionite test reagents allows an increase of light transmittance back to normal levels (green tracing). This reversion would not occur when non-S sickling hemoglobins induce the initial decrease in light transmittance.

movement. The hemoglobin will migrate at a rate determined by the net charge of the molecule, pH, ionic strength of the buffer and the type of supporting medium used.

Electrophoresis should not be considered definitive as a test to identify specific hemoglobin types. Many hemoglobins, although rare, have been reported to move like S under specified conditions of the test (Table C). Primary attention should be given to diagnosis of hemoglobin types potentially hazardous to the individual. Additional tests, such as the urea-dithionite test or other electrophoretic techniques (i.e. agar gel at pH 6.2), will indicate whether Hb S is involved. A combination of tests is most desirable whether solubility tests are used initially, or whether electrophoresis is used initially.

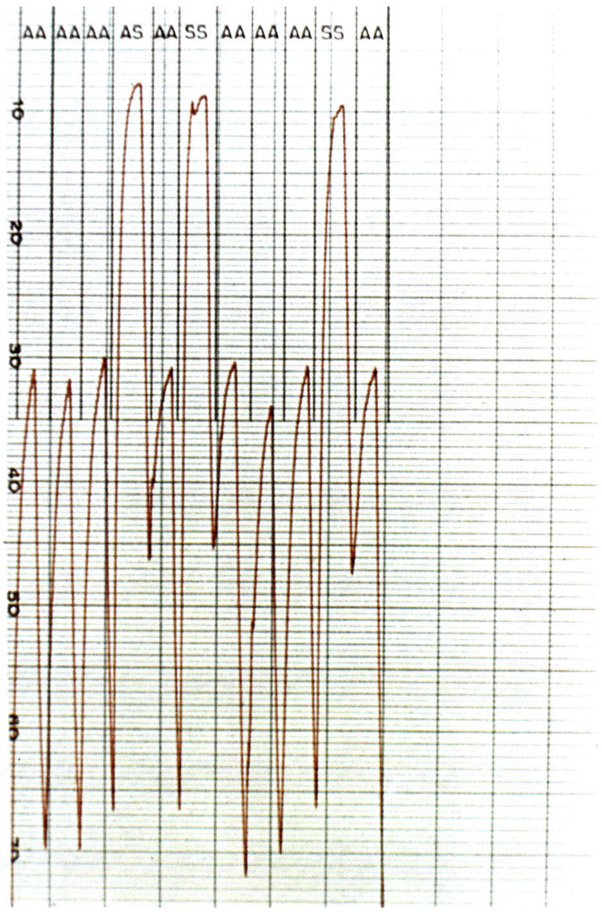

Figure 87. Amplification of automated dithionite test curves for ready identification of low solubility hemoglobins. Electrophoresis should be used in a second phase to distinguish S hemoglobin, non-S sickling hemoglobins, heterozygosities, and homozygosities.

Non-specificity of hemoglobin electrophoresis. Known abnormal hemoglobin, more rare than S, move like S under the usual pH ranges. Others have been reported to move like S under other electrophoretic conditions.

Table C
Hemoglobinopathies electrophoretically identical to hemoglobin S

At pH 8.0 to 8.9	Other specified conditions
S	Russ
D	Shimonoseki
Flatbush	Koln
Zurich	G (Philadelphia)
Stanleyville-II	G (Port Arthur)
Sealy (Sinai, Hasharon)	G (Galveston)
P	G (Texas)
Etobicoke	Alexandra
Sabine	Zurich
Gun Hill	E
Shimonoseki	Ocho Rios
Kokura	Kokura
UMI	UMI
Leiden	
L Ferrara	
Lepore	
G (Coushatta)	
Memphis/S	
Korle-Bu	
OSU-Christianborg	
Ocho Rios	

Many electrophoretic techniques are available with each possessing certain advantages and disadvantages. Most utilize stabilizing media, such as paper, agar, starch, starch-gel, cellulose acetate and acrylamide gel. Until recently most used *paper electrophoresis*. By this technique RBC hemolysates are applied to filter paper strips which are soaked in an electrolyte buffer at pH 8.6 and placed in a chamber in which an electric field is created. Advantages of zone electrophoresis on paper include low cost and simplicity; however the time required for optimal separation of the various hemoglobins is long, being about 20 hours.

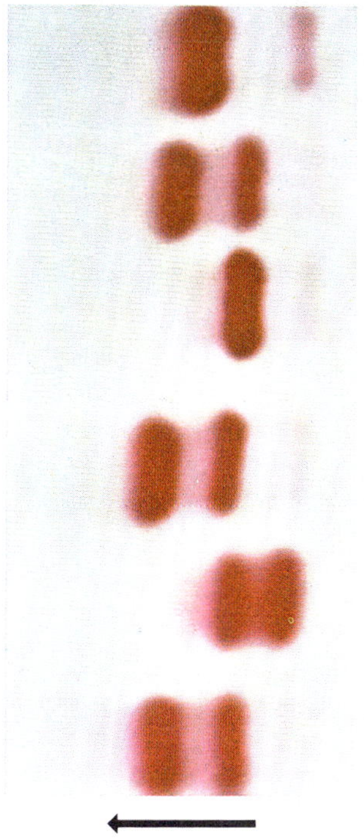

Figure 88. Hemoglobin electrophoresis on cellulose acetate.

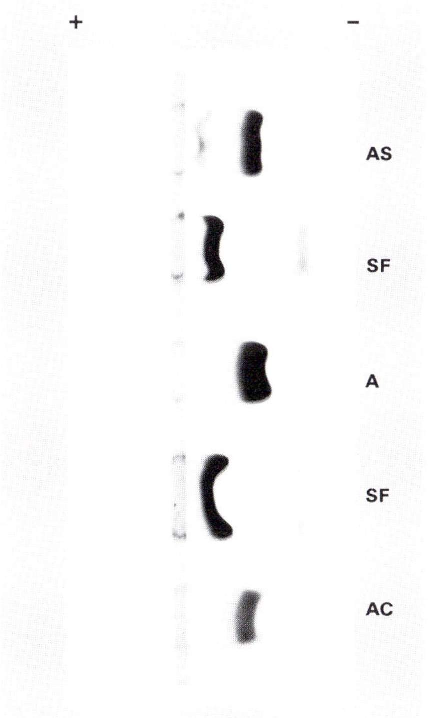

Figure 89. Separation of hemoglobins by electrophoresis on agar gel.

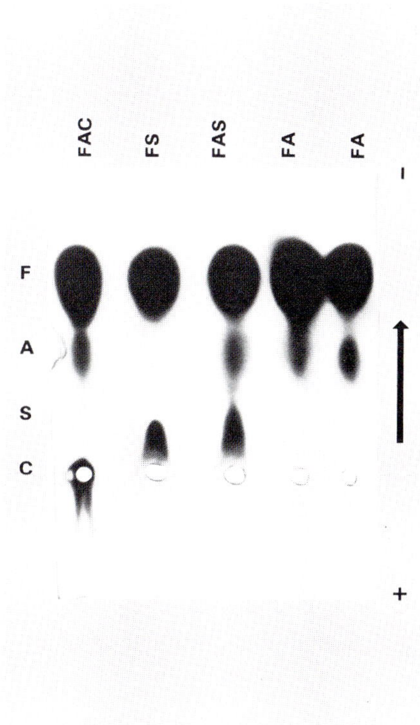

Figure 90. Agar gel electrophoresis of cord blood hemoglobin specimens. From top to bottom: hemoglobin C trait, sickle cell anemia, sickle cell trait, and specimens from two normal newborn infants.

Cellulose Acetate has gained increasing popularity as a supporting medium for hemoglobin electrophoresis. Its advantages over paper include rapid separation of hemoglobins (1-1/2 hours) and minimal adsorption of protein to the supporting material. In addition, this technique may be used for the diagnosis of thalassemia minor as definition is sufficiently clear to allow quantitation of Hb A_2. A micromethod employing a cellulose acetate medium for electrophoresis of capillary blood specimens has been employed on a large scale with excellent separation of many hemoglobin variants (Fig. 88).

Starch block electrophoresis has long been employed as the standard method for quantitating Hb A_2. After separation of the hemoglobin fractions by electrophoresis the starch block is cut and the various hemoglobin spots are removed. The hemoglobin is then eluted from the starch and measured spectrophotometrically.

Agar gel electrophoresis is somewhat time consuming but relatively simple to perform. It is particularly useful in separating Hb S from D. While these two abnormal hemoglobins have the same electrophoretic mobility on paper or cellulose acetate, in agar gel at pH 6.2, Hb D migrates with Hb A. Agar gel also allows complete separation of Hb F from adult hemoglobins (Fig. 89) and is the procedure of choice for the screening of neonates. It is capable of clearly differentiating between Hbs F, A, S and C in cord blood samples (Fig. 90).

Screening and Counselling

In considering a comprehensive screening program for hemoglobinopathies one's objectives must be clearly defined. Screening for sickle cell anemia is retrospective with implicit therapeutic overtones. Genetic counselling is prospective with preventive implications. Some view the main purpose of mass screening for sickle cell disease as identification of individuals with S hemoglobin in any form or combination. Others feel that mass screening should be designed to also identify hemoglobin C and perhaps other abnormal hemoglobins, gaining additional information for the purpose of genetic counselling and accumulation of statistics. Whether the emphasis is placed on identification of Hb S or on identification of hemoglobins S and C, such individuals must be provided with factual information so that they can make informed decisions regarding marriage and child bearing.

The optimal time for such screening is debatable but is probably in adolescence. The adolescent population is generally more readily accessible (as they are in school) for screening, education, and genetic counselling. Also such information will have greater relevance for this group.

No matter what age groups are being screened, testing should be voluntary and results kept confidential (i.e. given only to the individual or the family). In order to be well accepted and successful, any screening program for sickle cell must have the commitment and active participation of the Black

Table D
Illustrative gene combinations in selected hemoglobinopathies

	Parent (mother or father)	Genotypes (father or mother)	Percent genotype probability for each child					
			Homozygotes			Heterozygotes		
			AA	SS	CC	AS	SC	AC
Homozygotes								
	AA	AA	100					
	SS	SS		100				
	CC	CC			100			
	SS	AA				100		
	CC	SS					100	
	AA	CC						100
Homozygotes with heterozygotes								
	AA	AS	50			50		
	SS	AS		50		50		
	CC	SC			50		50	
	AC	SS				50	50	
	AA	SC				50		50
	CC	AS					50	50
Like heterozygotes								
	AS	AS	25	25		50		
	SC	SC		25	25		50	
	AC	AC	25		25			50
Unlike heterozygotes								
	AS	AC	25			25	25	25
	SC	AS		25		25	25	25
	SC	AC			25	25	25	25

community in all aspects of the program. Screening programs should be preceded by education in a non-alarming manner, and should be followed by education and genetic counselling.

It is particularly important that individuals involved be given a clear understanding of the differences between sickle cell anemia and sickle trait (Fig. 91 and Table D). An estimated two million American Blacks have the latter condition which is almost always completely benign. The individual found to have sickle trait should not be penalized in terms of life insurance rates, job opportunities,or participation in athletics as has unfortunately been done in some instances. The most important implication of sickle cell trait is a genetic one, for if both parents possess a gene for S hemoglobin, each of their offspring has a 1 in 4 chance of having sickle cell anemia (Fig. 91). Similarly if one parent has sickle trait and the other has C trait, each child has a 1 in 4 chance of having SC hemoglobinopathy (Fig. 91C).

AUTOMATED SCREENING

Attention in automated screening procedures is directed toward the individual with Hb S, who is most at risk. Hemoglobin C, either in the homozygote (CC) or heterozygote (AC),is considered innocuous and will not be detected in the initial phases. Difficulties arise when Hb C is combined with Hb S and these methods of mass screening emphasize the detection of Hb C only in this heterozygous condition. This is especially true during pregnancy when both the mother and the neonate are in serious risk of loss of life. Therefore, genetic counselling of the Hb S patient, with diagnostic studies of the spouse or proposed spouse for detection of S, C, thalassemia, or other disadvantageous hemoglobinopathies are recommended (Fig. 91 and Table D).

Mass screening programs should be designed to assure a low cost-to-effectiveness relationship with optimal diagnostic accuracy. Programs such as the "SCAT" (sickle cell anemia testing) program, a two-phase system, were designed by Nalbandian and associates. Emphasis is placed on detection of Hb S in any combination, detection of other low solubility hemoglobins, and detection of anemias in any form. Hemoglobin C is not given a position of primary importance unless present with S. The first phase utilizes the rapid, inexpensive, automated dithionite test. Screeners can expect to find approximately 10% of most U.S.A. Negro populations to have some combination of Hb S or some other low solubility hemoglobins. These positive specimens can then be subjected to electrophoresis and other sophisticated procedures for more precise identification of the hemoglobin abnormality. The designers of this program considered hemoglobin electrophoresis as nonspecific and relatively expensive to perform so that it is not used in the initial phase. Identification of some thalassemias and other anemias can be expected by use of this 2-phase screening method, by incorporating procedures capable of determining reduced hemoglobin levels or reduced mean corpuscular volume. Nichols has coupled automated hemoglobin level determination with automated dithionite testing for this purpose (Fig. 92). Phase 1 would then consist of the automated dithionite test coupled in tandem with hemoglobin level determination. Positive samples further tested by hemoglobin electrophoresis in Phase 2 would then detect homozygous S, heterozygous S, hemoglobin S combinations with other abnormal hemoglobins such as C, other potentially hazardous hemoglobinopathies such as M and alterations in levels of hemoglobin A_2 or F.

ELECTROPHORESIS FOR INITIAL SCREENING

Many others prefer hemoglobin electrophoresis for

Figure 91. Percentage odds for each genotype among progeny resulting from each pregnancy of parental matings SS X AA (**A**), SA X AA (**B**) and AS X AC (**C**). These 3 matings were selected as common and represent the 100, 50, and 25 percent odds situations.

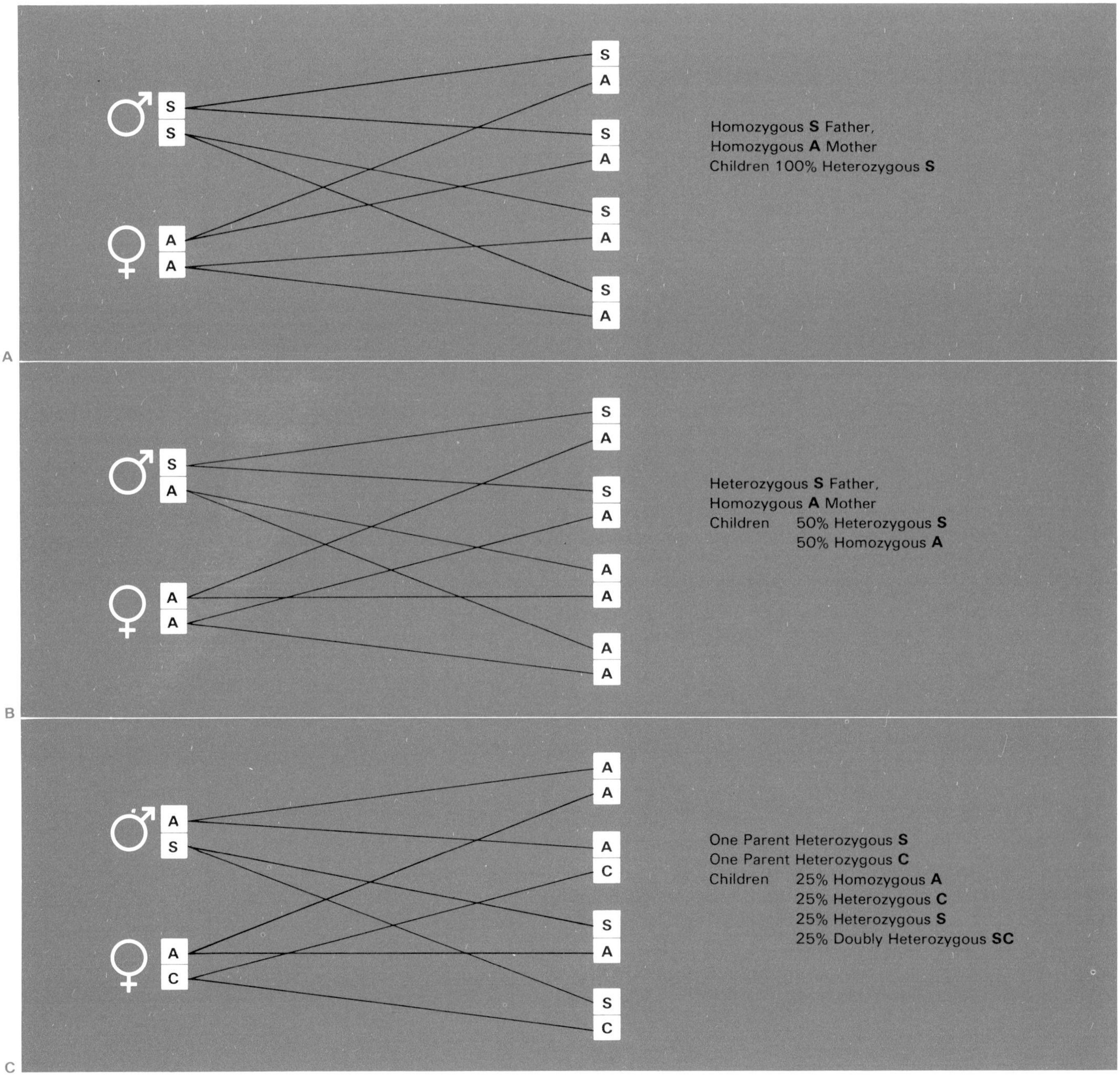

initial screening. Until recently this technique has been limited by the expense and the necessity of using venous blood. However, there are now rapid inexpensive electrophoretic methods which are applicable to mass screening programs. A micromethod employing cellulose acetate electrophoresis of capillary blood samples has been demonstrated to be quite reliable. Distinct bands clearly separate hemoglobins A, C and S, as well as A_2, allowing detection of some cases of β thalassemia trait. Those samples which contain abnormal hemoglobins should be then subjected to sickling and solubility tests (and additional testing in some instances, as agar gel electrophoresis at pH 6.2 if Hb D is suspected, and quantitation of hemoglobins A_2 and F to confirm a suspected diagnosis of β-thalassemia trait).

SCREENING AT BIRTH

The main objective of any screening program for sickle cell anemia is early diagnosis. If sickle cell anemia is diagnosed at birth or shortly thereafter the physician and parents can be alerted to the symptoms and signs of potentially serious complications, such as bacterial sepsis and aplastic crises. While sickling and solubility tests are unreliable in the first few months of life because of the high percentage of Hb F, one can make a definite diagnosis by agar gel electrophoresis at pH 6.2 as described by Robinson and Zuelzer.

Cord blood samples can be accurately screened as long as certain technical difficulties are understood. In the newborn the diagnosis of homozygous vs heterozygous S or Hb C is dependent on the recognition of small quantities of A, S and C in the presence of large amounts of F as differentiated by agar gel electrophoresis at pH 6.2 (Fig. 90). Paper electrophoresis is unsuitable because of its inability to separate Hb A from Hb F.

Figure 92. Typical curves obtained from a dual automated system for detection of sickling hemoglobins and anemia from any cause. The single black arrow (green curves) is for the automated dithionite tests. Note that specimens 76, 77, and 91 are positive for S hemoglobin (or some more rare sickling hemoglobin). The double arrow indicates curves for hemoglobin levels (red curves). Specimens 72 and 74 show that anemia is present.

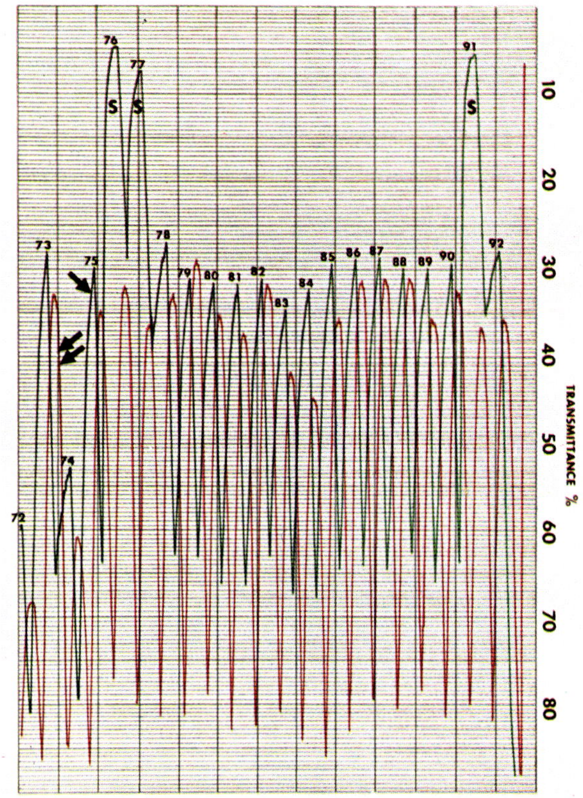

Treatment

Over the years treatment has been supportive and symptomatic only, attempting to alleviate pain or combat infections as they occur. We are now in the midst of an exciting era of promising research in sickle cell anemia and it seems probable that many poorly understood facets of the disease will be clarified and better methods of management will soon be available. Several promising agents are currently being evaluated and no doubt others will emerge.

While such investigational regimens are being devised and evaluated, what is considered the best available treatment for the individual with sickle cell anemia? Perhaps most important, those of us dealing with individuals with sickle cell anemia must have a good understanding of the disease and all of its complications. We must be constantly aware of the special problems presented by the sickle cell patient —their increased incidence of infections, their propensity to attacks of severe pain, necessitating narcotics in some instances. The patient and his family should also be given an understanding of the disease —what sort of things are likely to precipitate a pain crisis, and what to do when a pain crisis occurs. Also he or she should be made aware of the reasons for certain physical limitations, and what sort of activities and occupations they are better suited for, so that life can be fuller and more productive.

The two most common acute medical problems encountered are infection and pain crises. While pain may occur without obvious precipitating causes, infection is often associated with such vaso-occlusive episodes, especially in young children, and should be looked for.

MANAGEMENT OF PAIN CRISES

Symptomatic treatment of pain crises consists of analgesics and increased amounts of fluids. Fluids are quite important, since the patient in pain crisis is generally in negative fluid balance. This results from the following circumstances—the individual with sickle cell anemia has impairment of renal concentration and thus excretes large quantities of urine. In order to maintain adequate hydration, most consume large amounts of fluid. During a pain crisis, however, most patients *reduce* their fluid intake, and thus most are in NEGATIVE fluid balance when seen in the emergency room or other medical facility.

Pain crises vary considerably in frequency, duration, and intensity. Milder ones can usually be managed on an out-patient basis with increased amounts of oral fluids and analgesics such as aspirin, acetaminophen, propoxyphene hydrochloride, or codeine. Patients are instructed to increase their fluid intake as much as possible at the onset of a pain crisis and to take propoxyphene hydrochloride or aspirin at home and in some instances these measures are sufficient to alleviate pain. In pain crises characterized by pain, tenderness and local soft tissue swelling around joints or bone, some investigators have noted beneficial effects from certain anti-inflammatory agents.

When pain is severe and refractory to these measures, or if vomiting and dehydration supervene, hospitalization is necessary. Fluids are then given intravenously (I.V.) along with analgesic drugs such as codeine or meperidine. A variety of intravenous fluids (including electrolyte solutions, dextrose, dextran and plasma) have reportedly been effective in alleviating pain, presumably by their ability to mobilize trapped sickle cells. However, severe pain may persist for days or even weeks in some cases despite these measures.

MANAGEMENT OF BACTERIAL INFECTIONS

Because of the increased incidence of bacterial

infections, particularly overwhelming pneumococcal infection in children with sickle cell anemia, one should treat with antibiotics promptly when signs of infection develop. A child with sickle cell anemia who is seen in the emergency room with a temperature of 104° and slight dyspnea is at much greater risk than an otherwise normal child with similar findings. One should obtain appropriate cultures and institute antibiotic therapy immediately.

In the case of pneumonia, septicemia, meningitis or osteomyelitis the patient should also be transfused with packed cells to a hemoglobin of 11-12 gms %. Those seeing patients with sickle cell anemia should constantly keep in mind their propensity to bacterial infection—especially pneumococcal pneumonia.

Prophylaxis—What about pneumococcal vaccines? The pneumococcus is the most common offending organism in bacteremia and meningitis in sickle cell anemia, 80-85% of cases occurring in children under 3 years of age. Although a variety of serotypes of D. pneumoniae have been recovered, certain types seem more common than others (capsular types 1, 3, 6, 14, 18, 19, 23). While there is no epidemiologic evidence supporting the usefulness of polyvalent vaccines of pneumococcal capsular polysaccharides in children, their efficacy in preventing pneumococcal infection caused by specific serotypes in adults has been clearly demonstrated. From a theoretical standpoint active immunization of susceptible children seems desirable and certainly merits testing. The efficacy of immunization with suitably constituted polyvalent pneumococcal vaccines is currently being evaluated. Another unanswered question is whether such immunization might be followed by infections caused by other pneumococcal types in these children. Prophylaxis against infection during the seasons when respiratory infections are prevalent has been advocated by some but is not universally accepted.

PULMONARY INFARCTS

Vaso-occlusive episodes in certain areas require more specific therapeutic measures. In the case of a large pulmonary infarct, manifest by chest pain, dyspnea and fever, the roentgenogram picture is often indistinguishable from that of pneumonia, and in fact the two conditions may occur together. Blood and throat cultures should be taken, and in addition to I.V. fluids and antibiotics the patient should be transfused with packed cells to a hemoglobin of 11-12 gms %. The purpose of this is two-fold—the increased red cell mass will improve tissue oxygenation, and mixture of the sickled cells with normal red cells decreases blood viscosity. If the patient is moderately dyspneic oxygen should also be administered. In view of the high incidence of pneumococcal infections, penicillin is the antibiotic of choice until culture results are available.

CENTRAL NERVOUS SYSTEM INFARCTION

In the case of sudden vaso-occlusion involving the central nervous system (CNS) one is dealing with a medical emergency. If the involved blood vessel remains occluded for even a short time, infarction of that portion of the brain often results in permanent weakness, aphasia or convulsive disorder, or may even result in death. Attempts to mobilize stagnant cells must be immediate and should include infusion of large amounts of I.V. fluids, followed by blood transfusion as soon as possible. In addition, anticonvulsant medication—diazepam or phenobarbital—is given.

CNS infarction tends to be repetitive, i.e., an individual with sickle cell anemia who has had one or more episodes of CNS infarction is much more likely to have another such episode than a sickle cell anemia patient who has not had a CNS infarct. This no doubt reflects the progressive nature of large vessel occlusive disease (see p. 54), as well as greater vulnerability to hypoxia and stasis in an area where there has already been some circulatory compromise. In an attempt to prevent such recurrent episodes, we have had a group of children on a prophylactic transfusion program for the past 8 years. Each had a history of one or more episodes of CNS infarction which left them with permanent weakness and/or aphasia. Each is given 250-600 cc of buffy-poor packed cells (preceded by phlebotomy to reduce the risk of iron overload) every three weeks. In all, the percentage of hemoglobin A has been maintained over 75% and none has had an episode of CNS infarction, pain crisis or pneumonia while on this regimen. Several have had definite neurological improvement. However, one must always balance the beneficial effects against the known risks of multiple transfusions.

Individuals who have permanent neurologic deficits following CNS infarction often require specialized attention. The need for physiotherapy, speech therapy, occupational therapy must be individualized and should not be overlooked. "Maintenance" anticonvulsant medication may also be indicated in some.

MANAGEMENT OF HEMATOLOGIC CRISES

Aplastic Crises. Individuals with any type of chronic hemolytic anemia may have a sudden drop in hemoglobin resulting from a so-called "aplastic" (aregenerative) crisis. Such episodes usually occur in association with a viral infection and are characterized by a transient depression of erythropoiesis manifest by reticulocytopenia followed by a drop in hemoglobin—often to 2-3 gms %. While the aregenerative phase is self-limited (usually lasting 7-10 days), such dangerously low hemoglobin levels necessitate transfusion with packed cells to a hemoglobin of 6-8 gms % (Fig. 43).

Splenic Sequestration Crises. Sudden massive splenic sequestration of red cells may occur in infants or young children with sickle cell anemia without obvious precipitating cause. Often the child is brought in "D.O.A.", or is in shock from severe anemia (hemoglobin 1-2 gms %). In the latter situation, prompt diagnosis and treatment are essential for survival! Treatment should be directed at prompt correction of hypovolemia with plasma expanders followed by whole blood or packed cells as soon as possible. If shock can be reversed, dramatic regression of splenomegaly and return of sequestered blood to the general circulation often follow.

In view of the tendency to recurrent episodes of potentially life-threatening acute splenic sequestration, some recommend splenectomy for all survivors of an initial (or second) episode. Others prefer transfusing such children to hemoglobin levels of 11-12 gms %, and then maintaining their hemoglobin values above 10 gms % for the next several months with periodic packed cell transfusions. Although both approaches have obvious associated risks, the serious and recurrent nature of this complication would seem to justify consideration of either of these prophylactic measures.

RETINOPATHY

Proliferative retinopathy in SC and SS disease is a progressive disease, leading ultimately to vitreous hemorrhage, retinal detachment, and loss of vision (see p. 54 & p. 62). If seen early enough, the neovascular lesions can be prophylactically obliterated by photocoagulation, thus preventing progression of retinal damage.

PRIAPISM

Treatment of priapism in sickle cell anemia has been quite varied—both conservative and surgical methods have been recommended. The conservative management which we recommend consists of relief of pain and anxiety by the liberal use of analgesics and sedatives, plus transfusions with packed RBC to a hemoglobin of 11-12 gms %. Surgical methods have included aspiration of the corpora cavernosa with large bore needles, incision of the corpora, ligation of the dorsal arteries of the penis, and saphenocavernous shunting. The incidence of post-operative impotence and chordee is high, however, and it is our impression that medical management is preferable to surgical intervention.

LEG ULCERS

Among the numerous complications that may occur in sickle cell anemia, leg ulcers are particularly troublesome. Occurring predominantly in young adults, such ulcerations tend to become chronic and are often refractory to treatment. Management consists of bed rest, local measures to combat infection and promote healing, and packed cell transfusions. Despite these measures, ulcers may persist and skin grafting may be required. There is some evidence, although inconclusive, that oral zinc sulphate accelerates healing of these ulcers.

SURGICAL PROBLEMS

For the surgeon, sickle cell anemia poses a number of diagnostic as well as therapeutic problems. Acute abdominal pain crises, often accompanied by ileus, vomiting, fever, and leukocytosis, may be difficult to differentiate from acute appendicitis, acute cholecystitis or other surgical conditions.

When surgical intervention is necessary it may be performed relatively safely if certain precautions are rigidly observed. Preoperative transfusions, adequate hydration, and avoidance of hypoxia and acidosis are essential. Whenever possible, daily transfusions with packed RBC should be started one week pre-operatively, to attain a hemoglobin of 12-14 gms %. This will not only allow adequate time for equilibration within the cardiovascular system, but also results in temporary suppression of production of hemoglobin S RBC, thus further decreasing the percentage of circulating hemoglobin S RBC.

During anesthesia, hypoventilation may result in some degree of hypoxia and acidosis, which may lead to intravascular sickling, vaso-occlusion and infarction in the individual with sickle cell anemia. Cooling and stasis from positioning on the operating room table are additional factors which may enhance sickling. Dehydration and the use of tourniquets (as in certain orthopedic procedures) should also be avoided. During and after surgery the patient must be given adequate fluids and kept warm. In addition to the potential hazards of widespread intravascular sickling during anesthesia, patients with sickle cell anemia often present the additional problems of pre-existing changes within the heart, lung, liver, and kidney. When extensive, the latter may preclude an elective surgical procedure.

Postoperative morbidity is common, infections such as wound infections, pneumonia and bacteremia being the most frequent complications. Such infections should be looked for and treated promptly.

PREGNANCY

The pregnant patient presents special problems. By careful observation and immediate attention to seemingly minor problems, many potential complications can be avoided. Folic acid, 5-15 mgm daily, is recommended and may prevent a drop in hemoglobin values. (Iron, on the other hand, is unnecessary and will only lead to worsening of hemosiderosis.) Infections should be treated promptly and vigorously, and crises should be managed as previously outlined, with care given to maintenance of adequate hydration. Packed cell transfusions (or exchange transfusion using packed RBC) should be started between 30 and 34 weeks of gestation and continued intermittently to maintain an adequate level of hemoglobin (10-12 gms %). Such a transfusion program will also reduce the percentage of hemoglobin S RBC in the circulation, thus improving blood flow through small uterine and placental vessels. Labor and delivery should be undertaken with the patient in the best possible condition; i.e., with a hemoglobin above 11 gms %, free of infection, and well hydrated. Any anesthetic agents given should be carefully administered to avoid hypoxia and circulatory depression. The puerperium should also be carefully supervised, with attention to such potential complications as blood loss, infection, and phlebitis.

Patients with sickle cell anemia or SC disease should be counseled thoroughly regarding the advisability of pregnancy and its potential complications and risks. For those deciding against pregnancy, surgical sterilization should be offered. Another alternative, that of oral contraceptives, is at least theoretically objectionable from the standpoint of potential enhancement of thrombotic episodes, and some regard these agents as contraindicated in sickle cell anemia. SS and SC disease may also be indications for therapeutic abortion. However, each patient should be considered individually. The chronically ill and debilitated patient who already has multisystem involvement would obviously be a much greater obstetrical risk than the person with clinically mild disease.

INDICATIONS FOR BLOOD TRANSFUSION

There are relatively few indications for blood transfusion in sickle cell anemia. Hemoglobin levels tend to stabilize between 6-8 gms % and patients compensate to this degree of chronic anemia. However, packed cell transfusions are definitely indicated and may be lifesaving when there is a sudden drop in hemoglobin, such as occurs in an aplastic (aregenerative) crisis or with sudden splenic sequestration. Also in the case of pneumonia or pulmonary infarction or infarction of the central nervous system, transfusion with packed cells is often beneficial. In addition, leg ulcers tend to heal more rapidly when the hemoglobin level is maintained above 10 gms % with periodic transfusions of packed cells. Transfusions should also be given during the last trimester of pregnancy.

Another indication for blood transfusion is in preparation for surgical procedures where a general anesthetic will be used. When possible, patients should be transfused with packed cells to a hemoglobin of 12-14 gms % approximately one week preoperatively to allow equilibration within the cardiovascular system.

The beneficial effects of blood transfusion in sickle cell anemia may be summarized as follows: (1) the transfused RBC increase the oxygen-carrying capacity of the blood, thus promoting better oxygenation of tissues and (2) the transfused cells decrease the number and concentration of sickle cells (by dilution and by suppression of erythropoiesis) thus reducing blood viscosity and the tendency to stasis and vaso-occlusion. Risks to be considered include the possibility of transfusion reactions, serum hepatitis, and, in the case of multiple transfusions, hemochromatosis.

USE OF OXYGEN

Oxygen therapy has a very limited role in management of sickle cell anemia. It is generally of no value in alleviating pain crises, and is indicated only in the case of severe pneumonia or pulmonary infarction with dyspnea, or in the management of acute congestive heart failure. The latter usually results from a combination of severe anemia, myocardial weakness, and the additional stress of an infection such as pneumonia. In addition to oxygen, management consists of careful transfusion with small amounts (3 cc per pound of body weight) of packed cells (this may be preceded by phlebotomy) and digitalization with a cardiac glycoside.

INVESTIGATIONAL AGENTS

Thus far we have considered supportive and symptomatic treatment only, without attacking the basic problem, sickling of RBC, with resulting vaso-occlusion and infarction of tissues and organs. In this decade, treatment regimens have been designed to specifically prevent or reverse sickling of Hb S erythrocytes. The first of these investigational agents to show promise was *urea*. While many investigators have abandoned the use of this agent, feeling that it was ineffective in clinical situations, the use of urea represented the first ingenious attempt to treat the disease on a molecular level and thus is worthy of our attention.

Urea. The rationale for the use of urea in treating or preventing sickle cell vaso-occlusive episodes is based on Murayama's hypothesis that Hb S molecules, when deoxygenated, polymerize by means of hydrophobic interaction to form microfilaments and microcables resulting in distortion of the cell. Nalbandian postulated that any agent or condition diminishing hydrophobic interaction should interfere with the polymerization of Hb S tetramers, and thus prevent or reverse sickling. Although the RBC site(s) for urea action and exact mechanism as a desickling agent and inhibitor of sickling is still unresolved, urea action clearly differs from, and is independent of, cyanate. Urea in sugar solutions over a concentration range of 0.006 M—1.00 M blocks and reverses sickling of RBC. That the effect is due to urea per se is documented by Murayama's demonstration that urease treatment destroys the desickling effect of urea and has no effect on cyanate desickling. Subsequently, other physical chemists showed that similar concentrations of urea (0.005 M—1.0 M) reacted with experimental hydrogels (polymerized surgical implantation material) to increase water entry and holding within the gel. Of various agents studied *ex vivo*, urea seemed ideal in many respects. Urea is a small enough molecule to pass through the RBC membrane; it is metabolically inert, water soluble, nontoxic, and readily excreted. When given parenterally, however, urea must be infused in combination with sugars such as glucose or invert sugar to avoid hemolysis. The most undesirable property of urea is its potent diuretic action, making it potentially hazardous if fluid balance is not maintained.

Following a number of *ex vivo* observations (Fig. 93) clinical trials to determine the effectiveness of intravenous urea in invert sugar (U.I.S.) in alleviating severe pain crises were begun by Nalbandian and colleagues in 1970. Close supervision of such treatment was absolutely essential to avoid excessive diuresis and dehydration problems that would be life-threatening if uncontrolled. In most instances, urea seemed effective in controlling pain; however, all of these early studies were uncontrolled.

In 1973-74, several centers in the U.S. conducted randomized double-blind studies to evaluate the effectiveness of U.I.S. in the management of painful crises and concluded that this form of treatment was ineffective. (One should note, however, that none of these controlled trials used the precise regimen recommended by Nalbandian.) At any rate, it seems obvious that any such intermittent form of treatment is of limited usefulness, as it will have little or no

Figure 93. SEM comparison of a sickle-desickle cycle. **A.** Sickled RBC from Hb SS blood treated with metabisulfite to hasten deoxygenation. Note in this SEM field that there are only 3-4 typical biconcave discs. Also several extreme sickle forms with filamentous projections appear. **B.** The sickled RBC population illustrated by **A** were next treated with urea in glucose and a reversal of sickling occurred. Note many typical biconcave discs (about 10) resulted while sickle forms were reduced in number and also degree of sickling. (X 3800).

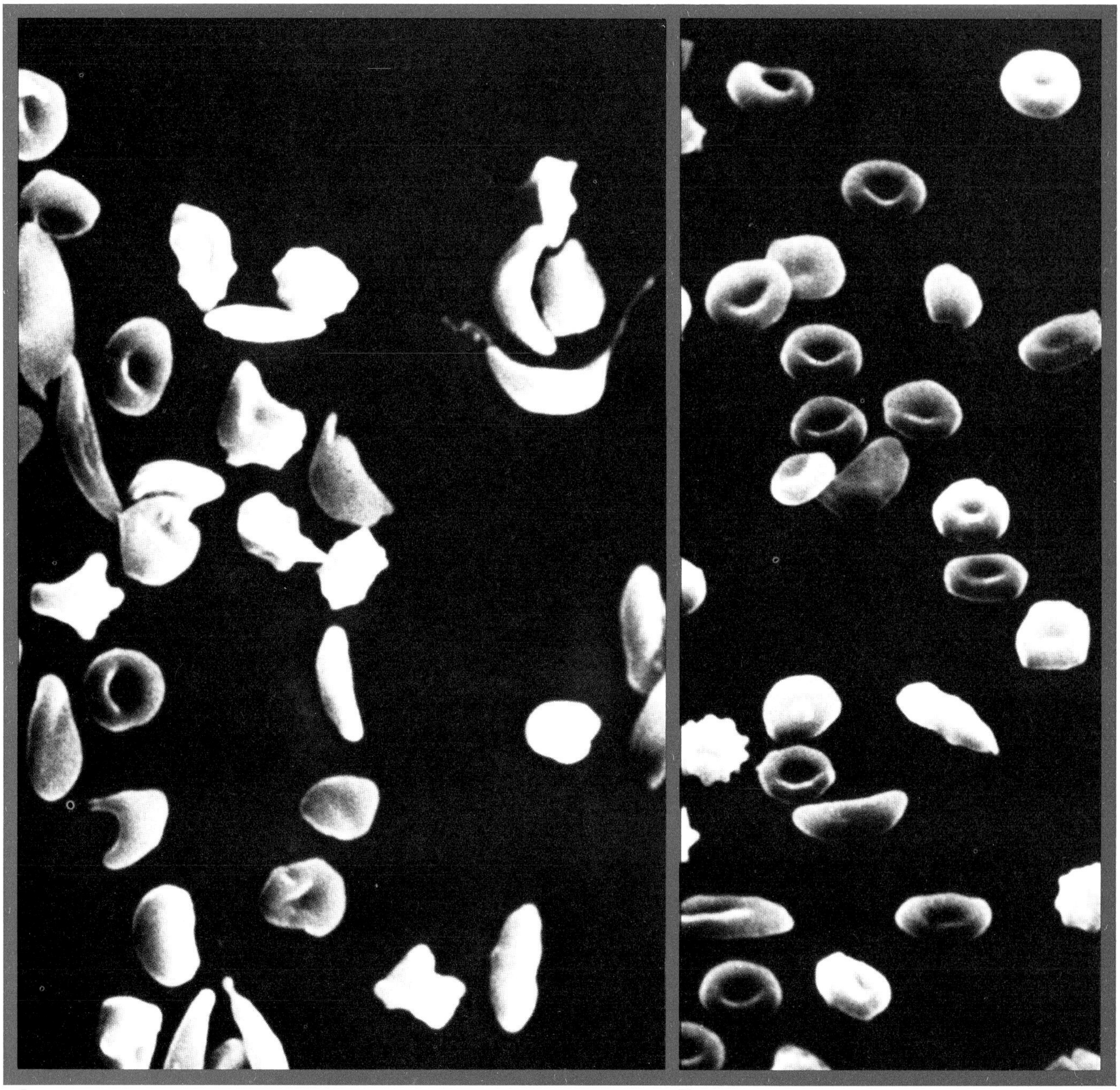

A B

effect in preventing the sequelae of less symptomatic episodes of vascular occlusion and infarction, with gradual loss of tissue and organ function, or in preventing the consequences of the chronic hemolytic anemia.

It thus seemed logical to attempt to prevent sickling by the daily administration of oral urea. If one could effectively prevent *in vivo* sickling, one should theoretically be able to prevent not only pain crises, but all of the devastating sequelae of the disease. A critical factor was the concentration of urea necessary to prevent or reverse sickling of Hb S erythrocytes. It was determined that as little as 0.006 M urea in glucose solution was capable of blocking sickling. This value corresponds to a blood urea nitrogen of 17 mgm %. The magnitude of sickling reversal is concentration-dependent, requiring somewhat higher concentrations (near 0.025 M, equivalent to a BUN of 70 mg %, well within a therapeutically attainable range) for reversal of 50% or more of sickled RBC.

In an attempt to evaluate the efficacy of daily oral urea "prophylaxis," a pilot study was begun at the Children's Hospital of Michigan in 1971-72. Twenty-one individuals with sickle cell anemia took oral urea for periods ranging from 3 to 12 months. There was significant reduction in the number of major vaso-occlusive episodes and infections in the group receiving oral urea, whereas no significant changes were noted in control subjects. This apparent clinical improvement could not be conclusively attributed to urea, as other factors may have played a role (such as the feeling of patients and their parents that something positive was being done for them).

Evaluation of any therapeutic modality in sickle cell anemia is exceedingly difficult because of the extreme variability in frequency, duration and intensity of pain crises, and because of the lack of objective criteria to determine the severity of vaso-occlusive episodes. In addition, reliability of results is dependent on whether the patient follows the prescribed dosage plan. When properly controlled regimens were followed, three-D evaluation of "circulating" red cells offered another objective parameter for clinical assessment. There was a significant reduction in the percentage of circulating sickle forms in urea-treated subjects (Fig. 94) but not in controls. Several other small-scale clinical studies of oral urea have been reported with varying approaches and controls. Conflicting results have been obtained. At any rate, in its presently available form, urea is inconvenient to take on a long-term basis. It is available only as a bulky, bitter-tasting powder and is rapidly excreted, necessitating frequent administration to maintain some elevation of blood urea nitrogen. For the above reasons, most investigators in the U.S. have now abandoned its use.

Figure 94. Percentage of normal biconcave disc forms in serial blood samples from one child with sickle cell anemia while on and off urea. Oral urea was started immediately following the initial blood sample (which contained 47% biconcave discs) and was discontinued 4 months later. Urea was restarted at 7 months.

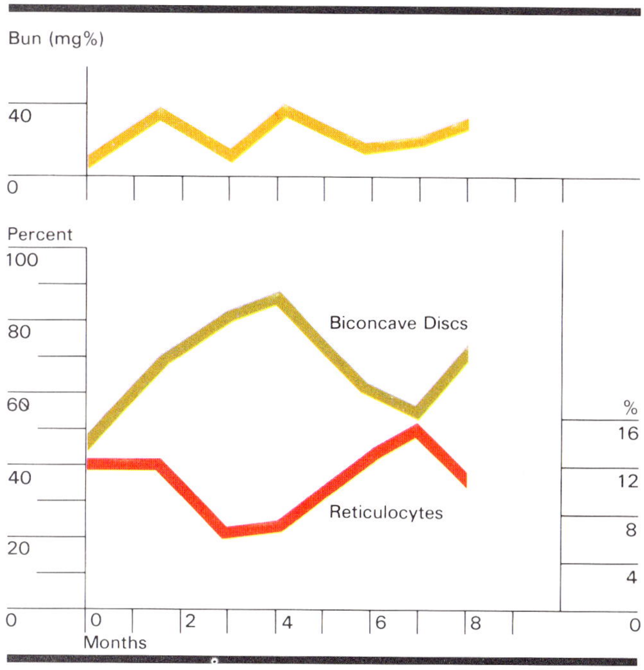

Cyanate. The next promising agent was potassium cyanate, proposed by Cerami and associates in 1971. The mechanism of action differs from that of urea. Potassium cyanate can effectively reduce the tendency of Hb S RBCs to sickle, but cannot reverse sickling that has already occurred. Cyanate action results primarily from increased oxygen affinity. Cyanate irreversibly carbamylates the N-terminal amino groups in α and β chains of oxygenated hemoglobin, resulting in a more electro-negative molecule. Thus an RBC whose Hb S molecules have once been carbamylated by cyanate is less likely to sickle, and this decreased tendency to sickle will persist throughout the cell's lifetime. The main reservation about the administration of cyanate was the potential carbamylation of other body proteins. It has been demonstrated that cyanate does react with many proteins and polypeptides in addition to hemoglobin, both *ex vivo* and *in vivo.* From 1973 through 1975, patient trials with oral sodium cyanate were conducted in several centers. No decrease in the number of painful crises was observed while patients were taking cyanate. Furthermore, a significant number of patients developed evidence of severe debilitating neurotoxicity, marked weight loss, and cataracts. (These posterior subcapsular lens opacities have occurred in individuals with normal G-6-PD as well as those with G-6-PD deficiency.)

While cyanate's toxicity thus precluded its further clinical use by the oral route, other investigators have tried weekly extracorporeal carbamylation of Hb S RBCs. While the number of patients studied to date is quite small, preliminary results suggest that the toxicity associated with oral administration of the drug is absent and that there may be a decrease in the number of pain crises as well as an increase in RBC survival. In ongoing studies, only the blood cells are exposed to cyanate, as the drug has deleterious effects on plasma proteins such as fibrinogen and complement as well.

Carbamyl Phosphate. Carbamylation of hemoglobin can also be achieved by carbamyl phosphate, an affinity labeling agent. According to Kraus and Kraus there is a difference in the extent of labeling of α and β chains with this agent. They found that α chains were preferentially labeled by ^{14}C carbamyl P while ^{14}C cyanate preferentially labeled the β chain. In addition to inhibiting sickling, incubation of homozygous S erythrocytes with carbamyl P has reportedly increased about two-fold the RBC survival as measured by ^{51}Cr. This agent is also undergoing further study.

SUMMARY

Treatment of sickle cell anemia over the years has been symptomatic and supportive. Severe pain crises have been treated with analgesic drugs and fluids, infections have been treated with antibiotics, but repetitive infarcts result in progressive deterioration of tissue and organ function. The devastating sequelae of this disease are not sufficiently altered by such symptomatic treatment.

We are now in a new era of molecular research in sickle cell anemia, and perhaps the greatest contribution of recent investigators has been to get us to look at sickle cell anemia in an entirely different way —to look at what actually takes place within the individual RBC, and to devise better methods of treatment aimed at altering molecular mechanisms. If the disease can be effectively attacked on this molecular level, preventing sickling, we should be able to prevent all of the clinical manifestations—the attacks of pain, the chronic anemia, the paralysis or weakness, infections and progressive disability so frequently seen in individuals with sickle cell anemia.

While our zeal for new and better methods of

medical management continues, we must not lose sight of the individual. Each has his or her special problems, anxieties and needs which must not be overlooked. Ideally an interested and efficient team of specialized personnel—including social worker, nurse, psychologist, physiotherapist, and others—should be available for guidance, coordination of care and activities, alleviation of fears and anxieties, and encouragement.

THE FUTURE

In this decade, the challenge of sickle cell anemia has been accepted and elevated in its priority as a major health problem. Chemotherapeutic attacks have been mounted at the abnormal molecule responsible for the devastating effects of sickling. However, treatment still remains symptomatic and supportive. No cure has been found for this hereditary disorder.

One promise of the future is that better therapy will result from the recent attention to the molecular defect. No doubt drugs superior to urea and cyanate will be found. Interruption or suppression of sickling or restriction of expression of the genetic defect should ultimately prevent all of the clinical manifestations of the disease. Thus the progressive disability, social and economic disadvantages, and reduced life expectancy should be prevented.

Health management teams should evolve to best serve the special interests and problems of the individual with sickle cell anemia. Physician, social worker, nurse, psychologist, genetic counselor, and others should be available for advice to the patient and family.

Another promise of the future lies in education to the realization that genetic imperfection should not be viewed as a stigma. Geneticists suggest that each individual most likely carries 5 to 10 potentially harmful genes that may be expressed during one's lifetime or passed to offspring. Thus we must learn to deal with expressed genetic defects to minimize their activation or interaction with environmental factors. Education should ensure that people with sickle cell trait should not be penalized now or in the future by job discrimination or insurance deprivation.

In addition, informed bearers of genetic defects have some options concerning marriage, child bearing, or pregnancy termination as well as improving circumstances for their afflicted children. While genetic engineering is talked about, we seem far from practical solutions to repair gene defects even should this be deemed ethical. An exciting development is the prospect that fetal blood sampling can provide data to identify sickle cell anemia or other genetic disorders as early as the 17th week of pregnancy. This new pregnancy testing procedure does not yet deserve the acceptance given to amniocentesis as a forecaster of severe genetic defects. In the future, however, parents may be able to make realistic decisions on whether or not to terminate a pregnancy when the fetus has a disastrous type of hemoglobinopathy.

A further promise of the future is that rapid, specific and inexpensive screening methods coupled with education and counseling will be widely available although not mandatory. The main advantages are 1) early detection of sickle cell anemia for medical management or prevention of the deleterious consequences of sickling and 2) acquisition of genetic information for family planning.

Appendix

CLINICAL AND LABORATORY FEATURES OF SELECTED HEMOGLOBINOPATHIES.

Genotype	Anemia	Splenomegaly	Other Clincal Features	Peripheral Blood Smear	Sickling Tests	Clinical Severity	Remarks
AS	None	No	Usually none	Normal	Positive	None	May have hematuria. Generally problems occur under unphysiologic conditions.
SS	Severe	Yes, but uncommon after childhood.	Intermittent pain crises. Bone and joint infarcts. Increased bacterial infections.	Sickle forms, target cells, hypochromia, polychromasia.	Positive	Severe	Progressive disability common. Shortened life span.
SC	Mild to moderate	Common	Intermittent pain crises. Bone and joint infarcts (less common than in SS). Retinopathy common in adults.	Aniso—and poikilocytosis, target cells, hypochromia, polychromasia.	Positive	Mild to moderate	Severity often increased during pregnancy. Intracellular crystals.
S-β-Thal	Moderate to severe	Occasional	Intermittent pain crises. Bone and joint infarcts.	Aniso—and poikilocytosis, target cells, hypochromia, polychromasia.	Positive	Moderate to severe	May have no Hb A or subnormal amount.
CC	Mild to moderate	Occasional	Usually none.	Many target cells, spherocytes.	Negative	Mild	Intracellular crystals.
DS	Mild to moderate	Common	May have arthralgia. Abdominal pain.	Sickle forms, target cells, polychromasia, nucleated RBC.	Positive	Mild to moderate	Should be considered if clinical manifestations unusually mild for SS. D may be distinguished from S by agar gel at acid pH.
OS	Severe	Yes, but uncommon after childhood.	Similar to SS (more severe than SC disease).	Sickle forms, target cells, hypochromia, polychromasia.	Positive	Moderate to severe	May be mistaken for SC. Distinguish by agar gel electrophoresis at acid pH.
ES	Mild	No	Usually none.	Hypochromia, microcytosis.	Positive	Mild	Found among Eti-Turks.
Heterozygous β-Thal	Mild to moderate	Occasional	Usually none.	Hypochromia, microcytosis, target cells, slight polychromasia.	Negative	Mild	Peripheral blood film resembles mild iron deficiency anemia. Elevated Hb A_2 and F Diagnostic.
E-Thal	Severe	Common	Gradual development of hemochromatosis, congestive heart failure, hepatic dysfunction.	Hypochromia, target cells, Anisopoikilocytosis and poikilocytosis, nucleated RBC.	Negative	Moderate to severe	Shortened life span; often complicated by parasitism and other infections.

SELECTED READING LIST

(Also see references in acknowledgement list)

Books and Monographs

1. Abramson, H., Bertles, J. F., and Wethers, D. Eds.: Sickle Cell Disease, diagnosis, management, education and research. (Symposium Proceedings, N.Y., Nov., 1971) C. V. Mosby Co., St. Louis, 1973.

2. Greenwalt, T. J. and Jamieson, G. A.: *Formation and Destruction of Blood Cells.* Lippincott, Philadelphia, 1970.

3. Harris, J. W. and Kellermeyer, R. W.: *The Red Cell (Production, Metabolism, Destruction: Normal and Abnormal).* Revised Edition. Commonwealth Fund, Harvard Univ. Press, Cambridge, Mass., 1970.

4. Jonxis, J. H. P. and Huisman, T. H. J.: *A Laboratory Manual on Abnormal Hemoglobins.* 2nd Ed., Blackwell Scientific Publications, Oxford & Edinburgh, 1968.

5. Livingston, F. B.: *Abnormal Hemoglobins in Human Pathology.* Aldine Publ., Chicago, 1967.

6. Mammen, E. F., Anderson, G. F. and Barnhart, M. I., eds.: Sickle Cell Disease. (Proceedings 20th Annual Symposium on Blood, Jan., 1972, Wayne State Univ. Sch. Med., Detroit.) *Thrombos. Diath. Haemorrh. Supp.*, 1973.

7. Murayama, M., and Nalbandian, R. M.: *Sickle Cell Hemoglobin: Molecule to Man.* Boston, Mass., Little Brown and Co., 1973.

8. Nalbandian, R. M. (ed): *Molecular Aspects of Sickle Cell Hemoglobin, Clinical Applications,* Springfield, Ill., Charles C. Thomas, 1971.

9. World Health Organization Technical Report Series No. 338, 1966 and No. 509, 1972. Pub. World Health Organization, Geneva.

Individual Citations

1. Allison, A. C.: Genetic Factors in Resistance to Malaria. *Ann. N. Y. Acad. Sci.* 91: 710-729, 1961.

2. Cerami, A., Manning, J. M., Gillette, P. N., De Furia, F., Miller, D., Graziano, J. H., and Peterson, C. M.: Effect of Cyanate on Red Blood Cell Sickling. *Fed. Proc.* 32: 1668-1672, 1973.

3. Diggs, L. W.: Sickle Cell Crises. *American Journal of Clinical Pathology* 44: 1-19, 1965.

4. Harkness, D. R. and Roth, S.. Clinical Evaluation of Cyanate in Sickle Cell Anemia. *Prog. Hematol.* 9: 157-184, 1975.

5. Herrick, J. B.: Peculiar elongated and sickle-shaped red blood corpuscles in a case of severe anemia. *Arch. Int. Med.* 6: 517-521, 1910.

6. Henry, R., Nalbandian, R., Nichols, B., Wolf, P., Camp, F. Jr., and Conte, N.: An Automated Specific Method for the Detection of S Hemoglobin. *Advances in Automated Analysis.* Vol. I, Edited by E. C. Barton, et al., Thurman Associates, Miami, Fla., 1971. pp. 471-476.

7. Johnston, R. B., Newman, S. L. and Struth, A. G.: An Abnormality of the Alternate Pathway of Complement Activation in Sickle Cell Disease. *New England Journal Medicine* 288: 803-808, 1973.

8. LaCelle, P. L. and Weed, R. I.: The Contribution of Normal and Pathologic Erythrocytes to Blood Rheology, In *Prog. Hematol.* Ed. E. B. Brown and C. V. Moore. Vol. VII Grune & Stratton, 1971, pp. 1-31.

9. Lukens, J. N.: Hemoglobin S, the Pneumococcus and the Spleen. *Am. J. Dis. Child.* 123: 6-7, 1972.

10. Lusher, J. M. and Barnhart, M. I.: Evaluation of Oral Urea in the Management of Sickle Cell Anemia. *In* Hemoglobin and Red Cell Structure and Function (Proceedings 2nd Internat. Conf. On Red Cell Metabolism & Function, Univ. Mich., Ann Arbor, Apr., 1972). Ed. G. J. Brewer, Plenum Press, New York, 1972.

11. Neel, J. V.: The Clinical Detection of the Genetic Carriers of Inherited Disease. *Medicine* 26: 115-153, 1947.

12. Pauling, L., Itano, H. A., Singer, S. J., and Wells, I. C.: Sickle Cell Anemia, A Molecular Disease. *Science* 110: 543-548, 1949.

13. Perutz, M. F.: Structure and Function of Hemoglobin. I. A. Tentative Atomic Model of Horse Hemoglobin. *J. Molec. Biol.* 13: 646-668, 1965.

14. Perkins, R. P.: Inherited Disorders of Hemoglobin Synthesis and Pregnancy. *Am. J. Ob. Gyn.* 111: 120-159, 1971.

15. Robinson, A., Harrison, A. and Zuelzer, W. W.: A New Technique for Differentiation of Hemoglobin, *J. Lab. & Clin. Med.* 50: 745-752, 1957.

16. Schwartz, A. D. and Pearson, H. A.: Impaired Antibody Response to Intravenous Immunization in Sickle Cell Anemia. *Pediat. Res.* 6: 145-149, 1972.

17. Stamatoyannopoulas, G.: The Molecular Basis of Hemoglobin Disease. *Ann. Rev. of Genetics.* 47-70, 1972.

18. Walsh, R. T., Lusher, J. M. and Barnhart, M. I.: Coagulation and Fibrinolysis Studies in Sickle Cell Disease. *Thrombos. Diathes. Haemorr. Supp.* 53: 171-181, 1973.

19. Weiss, L., and Tavassoli, M.: Anatomical Hazards to Passage of Erythrocytes through the Spleen. *Sem. Hematol.* 7: 372-381, 1970.

20. White, J. G.: The Fine Structure of Sickled Hemoglobin *in situ. Blood.* 31: 561, 1968.

21. Yawson, G. I., Huntsman, R. G. and Metters, J. S.: An Assessment of Techniques Suitable for the Diagnosis of Sickle Cell Disease and Haemoglobin C Disease in Cord Blood Samples. *J. Clin. Path.* 23: 533-537, 1970.

ACKNOWLEDGEMENTS

Figure 1. Precision scale model was constructed by Dr. Makio Murayama of the National Institutes of Health, Bethesda, MD from the atomic coordinates determined by Dr. Max Perutz, Cambridge, England.

Figures 6, 7, and 8. Reproduced and modified by permission from R. M. Nalbandian, R. L. Henry, F. R. Camp, Jr., P. L. Wolf and T. N. Evans, *Obstet. Gynec. Survey* 26: 185-191, 1971.

Figure 17. Dr. Flossie Cohen, Dept. Pediatrics, Wayne State University School of Medicine, Detroit, MI.

Figure 29. Dr. Per-Ingvar Branemark. *Intravascular Anatomy of Blood Cells in Man,* Karger, New York, NY, 1971.

Figures 38 and 44. Dr. Ruth A. Seeler, Abraham Lincoln School of Medicine, Chicago, IL.

Figure 48. Dr. J. O. Reed, Children's Hospital of Michigan, Detroit, MI.

Figure 55. Dr. Arnold Axelrod, Dept. of Internal Medicine, Wayne State University School of Medicine, Detroit, MI.

Figure 57. Dr. L. W. Statius van Eps, C. Pinedo-Veets, G. H. DeVries, and J. de Koning, Jr., *Lancet* 1: 450-452, 1970.

Figure 62. Dr. Morton F. Goldberg, *Arch. Ophthal.* 85: 428-437, 1971.

Figures 68, 69, and 70. Reproduced and modified from art reference by Dr. C. A. Baechler, Dept. Physiology, Wayne State University School of Medicine, Detroit, MI.

Figures 71, 72, 74, 78, and 83. Dr. R. M. Nalbandian, ed., *Molecular Aspects of Sickle Cell Hemoglobin: Clinical Applications.* Charles C. Thomas, Springfield, 1971.

Figures 73, 75, 76, 79, 80, 81, and 82. Dr. M. Murayama and R. Nalbandian. *Sickle Cell Hemoglobin: Molecule to Man.* Little Brown & Co., Boston, 1973.

Figures 83 and 84. R. M. Nalbandian, B. M. Nicols, F. R. Camp, Jr., J. M. Lusher, N. F. Conte, R. L. Henry, and P. L. Wolf. *Clin. Chem.* 17: 1028-1032, 1971.

Figures 85, 86, and 87. R. M. Nalbandian, B. M. Nicols, F. R. Camp, Jr., J. M. Lusher, N. F. Conte, R. L. Henry and P. L. Wolf. *Clin. Chem.* 17: 1033-1037, 1971.

Figure 89. Dr. Y. Ravi, Child Research Center of Michigan, Detroit, MI.

Figure 90. Dr. H. A. Pearson and R. T. O'Brien. *J. Pediat.* 81: 1201-1204, 1972.

Figure 92. Dr. B. M. Nichols and E. L. Bemis. *In* U. S. Army Med. Res. Lab. Report No. 1014, 16 Jan., 1973.

Figure 94. Dr. J. M. Lusher and M. I. Barnhart. *In* Hemoglobin and Red Cell Structure and Function, G. J. Brewer, ed., Plenum Press, New York, 1972.